I dedicate this book to my Uncle Bill. He was my knight in shining armor, but I never got to thank him properly. He passed away in 2023 and left a hole in our hearts.

RIP, Uncle Bill. We love you.

Driven by the pursuit of perfection and the desire to truly be loved and accepted, Cynthia battled an eating disorder for thirteen long years.

"Starving, Bingeing, Purging" is her raw, authentic story, told firsthand; a story not just of suffering, but of resilience, victory, and hope against all odds.

~Fatima Aladdin, master's degree in
English Language and Literature

"Starving, Bingeing, Purging-the true story of how I recovered from an eating disorder-and you can too! by Cynthia Star, is a remarkably candid and beautifully written book that EVERYONE can benefit from reading. These are valuable life lessons and Cynthia Star's book- Starving, Bingeing, Purging- should be mandatory reading for every student in high school. It IS that good."

Diane Klein, Publisher
- Across the Pond Publications

Starving, Bingeing, Purging

The true story of how I recovered from an eating disorder- and you can too!

CYNTHIA STAR

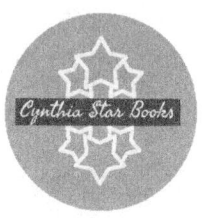

Published by Cynthia Star Books

www.cynthiastarbooks.com

Copyright 2024 by Cynthia Star

Contact:
Facebook/CynthiaStarBooks.com@cynthiastarbooks

Edited by: Bruce Welton

ISBN: 979-8-9850681-7-7

Also, by Cynthia Star

The Beepy Bumpy Blue Bug
~ picture book (ages 2-6)

What Color is Your Dragon?
~ picture book (ages 4-8)

The Moonlit Dragon
~ picture book (ages 4-8)

The Dragon Flyers Book One
~ (ages 7-10)

The Dragon Flyers Book Two
~ (ages 7-10)

The Dragon Flyers Book Three
~ (ages 7-13)

The Dragon Flyers Book Four
~ (ages 8-13)

Happiness Came with a Cat (New Edition)
~ Adult memoir/self-help

Contents

Introduction

I've spent the last couple of years thinking about writing this book. I've talked myself out of it several times because, to write this story, I would have to dig deep into my past. I would have to be honest, raw, and expose myself. That exercise would be difficult for someone who once hid from every emotion, feeling, and truth. I lied to myself and hid from other people because the truth was too hard for me to face, so I avoided it at all costs. I finally decided to write this account of my life dealing with eating disorders, though, because I knew someone out there needed to hear what I had to say: a family member, a doctor, a friend, or someone suffering with an eating disorder. I hope this book will help you to understand the struggles around this illness- and to find hope.

Are you the person locked in the pit of hell with what seems like no escape? This book is for you.

Do you believe that recovery is impossible? Do you hate yourself? This book is for you.

Have you lost all hope of being able to recover? Then let me give you my hope, my happiness, and my belief that you can do it- until you believe it for yourself.

Because you believe what you tell yourself. Your mind doesn't know if what you are saying is truth or not. What you feed your mind manifests itself in your body. And the body keeps score. You have fed yourself lies and your body believed you. You have hidden as I did from what is eating you inside.

Will you be brave and take this journey with me? Will you allow me to be vulnerable for you? Will you let me feel things for you- at least until you can feel them yourself and be ok with them?

Let me carry the burden you are dragging around.

If you are a parent, a friend, a counselor or lover of someone with an eating disorder, will you be brave for the person with an eating disorder until they can be brave for themselves?

Do you believe that you are part of the solution? What if you are part of the problem? And if you are part of the problem, what can you do?

In these pages, I'm going to share my story- about when and where my eating disorder started, and what I felt, thought, and did while amidst the darkness. I'm going to tell you what I told myself, how I felt, how I thought. If you are ready for the raw truth, then read on. There is power in my story that can free you or a loved one. If you are part of the problem, you may recognize yourself in this book.

My hard-won lessons over the last sixty years have led me to write this book. I share my struggles, my pain, my fears, and finally how I gained freedom from the chains that bound me- and how you can, too.

Tears fill my eyes and I weep as I type these words- because I can feel your pain, your burden, and the things you hide from, as I once did. At first, I thought I was feeling my pain, but I realized that these tears were not shed for me. They are shed for you.

>)•(<

PART ONE

>)•(<

ONE:

It starts Childhood years

I remember sitting at the table, swinging my legs, staring at the plate of eggs in front of me. I was alone. Everyone else had left the room a long time ago. Everyone, except me. I couldn't leave until I ate the eggs. I hated eggs, yet here they sat on my plate, staring at me with big yellow eyes. Bacon, I liked. Cereal, I liked. Pancakes, I liked. But not eggs.

Then why did I have to eat them? Because my mom said I had to. The same way I had to eat spinach (which I still don't like), and liver and onions. Back in the 1960s when I was growing up, it was *the way*. You ate what was put on your plate and you were grateful. By God, there were people starving in third world countries and you should be grateful. That was how my parents and grandparents were raised. No one questioned it. They passed it on from generation to generation. Reacting to that rule is where the battles over food began, pitching my iron will against my mom's.

She was tough, but I could outlast her. I knew eventually that she'd let me off of that chair and I'd run away to play. I hated eggs more than I hated an empty stomach or sitting there for hours, playing with the cold food on my plate. That's all it was for me: a simple truth. I don't like eggs or liver or onions, so I will not eat them, and you can't make me.

When you're a kid, your tastebuds must differ from those of adults. Children either have unsophisticated tastebuds, or their tastebuds are more sensitive to bitter, sweet, and sour, which magnify flavorings. At least, that's my theory. I still don't like eggs very much; I can't eat them without ketchup or toast and jam or bacon or ham. And liver, nope, I still think it's gross.

In keeping me at the table until I finished my food, causing harm was not my mom's intention. I was to learn later in life that my mom had suffered much more than I did enduring physical abuse by her dad. She was a survivor, a victim herself of misguided parental law.

It's amazing to me how powerful food is. A food's taste, smell, or texture can evoke emotions, good or bad, depending on what our early experience with it entailed.

Welch's grape juice is like that for me. If I smell it- or even see the bottle, I'm transported back to my childhood, sitting on my dad's lap as he eats breakfast. There is a glass of grape juice, a half of a grapefruit covered with sugar, two pieces of buttered toast, and a bowl of cornflakes in front of us. He lets me sip his grape juice and feeds me bites of cereal as he balances me on his lap and tries to finish his breakfast. Food never tasted so good. No matter how many years go by, one whiff of Welch's grape juice evokes this memory. And it is bittersweet.

I cherish that moment of being with my dad, his powerful arms holding me, a purple mustache on my lips. If only I could have stayed the little girl, resting on my daddy's knee, happily sipping juice as he fed me bites of soggy cereal. I also see the juice glass empty in front of me and it reminds me of all I lost, and of the personal emptiness I sought to fill for the next thirty years with his absence. I loved my dad so much. Much more than he loved me.

My relationship with my father in his later years was tumultuous. My relationship with food was like that, too. I tried to fill the hole his absence left in my heart by micromanaging my diet. But that hole was so deep, no amount of starving, bingeing or purging ever filled the space.

It would be many years before I accepted the hard truth that he would never be what I needed. I continued to suffer, using food as a crutch for control and comfort, until I realized that he loved me as much as he was able, which was far short of what I needed.

When he passed two years ago, I hardly felt a thing. I never went to his funeral or received anything that belonged to him, and I never asked for anything, because so many years had gone by without him being there, and I no longer cared.

He was not the dad I had needed, no matter how hard I had wished he might be- until I no longer wanted him.

There were many hard lessons I was to learn in life, and it would be a very long time before I could handle them healthily.

TWO:

In the shadows

When I was young, I grew up in a middle-class family of five in small-town Nebraska. I had two older brothers, and we were each two years apart. I was the only girl and the baby of the family, which turned out to be a blessing and a curse. As a girl with two older brothers, it's no wonder I later became a tomboy. Boy-stuff was all I knew, so becoming a tomboy fit a natural progression.

My dad grew up in a big farm family with ten brothers and sisters, and maybe that's why he was so aloof and selfish. Among that many children, perhaps he was just one of the herd- another strong back for labor, another mouth to feed, or even another inconvenience. I don't recall my dad talking much about life on the farm or what it was like growing up in such a big family, but I remember visiting the farm and enjoying spreads of food on my grandmother's long wooden table: homemade bread, freshly churned butter, thick slices of meat with mashed potatoes and brown gravy, cherry or apple pie for dessert.

The Sunday noon meal at the farm was not just a meal- it was an experience. Food passed around that table like a friendly conversation. Smelling the savory scent of roast beef, and seeing heat curls rise above the gravy that pooled in the buttery mounds of mashed potatoes on my plate were some of my fondest memories of visiting the farm. Those, and visiting the horses. Like most young girls, I dreamed of having a horse and I was obsessed with them. I drew horses, read about horses, pretended to be a horse, played with toy horses, and begged for one.

So, of course, whenever we visited the farm, I wanted to ride a horse. Grandpa would take me out to the barn and show me the cattle, the chickens, the hogs, and tease me about riding the bull.

"No grandpa, I want to ride a horse. Pleeease, grandpa."

Young me knew that he had horses because I'd seen them out in the pasture. There were telltale bridles, halters and harnesses hanging on the barn wall, so there was no fooling me. Grandpa had horses, and I wanted to ride one. What I didn't understand was that the horses he had were large plow horses, used only for work. A working farm had no place for animals that didn't produce. With so many mouths to feed, there was no time or money for a pleasure horse to ride simply for fun. But I was too young to understand that.

I was to be disappointed every time we visited the farm, but I never stopped begging. When you're a kid, it's ok to beg. There's no pride stopping you, so you just keep asking, no matter how many times a grown up tells you no. So I kept asking- at least until we stopped visiting the farm when my parents separated.

My connection with food on the farm had been pleasant, until it was gone, along with my dad.

Divorces were harder, and took longer, to get in the '60s. I guess they gave you time to reconcile before signing the final papers, and the waiting period almost worked. At one point, my mom told us that she and my dad were getting back together. That was great news to me, and I remember feeling excited, until we spent a weekend camping with my dad.

He brought his girlfriend and her spoiled brat daughter. We knew she was his girlfriend because at night when they thought we were sleeping, we would hear them whispering from the bed in the back of the airstream trailer.

"Stop it, Harold. The kids are here," she said.

"Oh, come on, just a little fun?" Dad said.

"No," she said, giggling and slapping his hand.

And so it went that weekend, the cat-and-mouse game my dad played with her. I was too young to process the information. How could this be happening? Mom and Dad were married. They were getting back together, right?

We told mom about the trip as soon as we saw her. Soon after that, we had the next serious family conversation that changed our lives.

It was also the conversation where I learned that my voice didn't matter. No one meant it that way at the time, and I didn't understand the impact it would have on my life until many years later, but now that I'm an adult, I understand the significance of the conversation. It was then that I learned that what I had to say wasn't important.

We were riding in the car. Mom was driving while talking to the three of us, probably smoking a cigarette, as was her habit.

"She's pregnant," mom said. "Bonnie is pregnant."

She let that one soak in. Bonnie was dad's girlfriend. There it was, the words that changed our lives. But what happened next is the part that still disturbs me.

"What do you all think?" mom asked. "What should we do?"

Moms raising kids alone have a unique relationship with their children. In the absence of a partner, sometimes mothers discuss things with their kids that normally they wouldn't because her relationship dynamics change without a mate, and mother and children become survivors together. It's them against the world. In dysfunctional families, children may become confidants when parents cross personal boundaries. A parent may treat them more like partners than children. At least, that's what happened in our family. And the more dysfunction exists, the more boundaries people cross.

Somehow, we kids understood that what my mom (or we) decided about this situation would determine the future- for us, and for the baby. Either we kept our dad for ourselves, or we let his new family have him. Or more accurately, we let the baby have him.

I don't recall the rest of the conversation- just its outcome, and the shock I felt. It was determined that the baby needed dad more than we did. What? We were his family, not them! We were here first! Didn't we matter? Don't three children trump one? Aren't my parents still married and she's just the girlfriend? The injustice of the situation hit me. Even as a young child, I understood the unfairness. But everyone agreed that the baby needed him more than we did. Except for me. I didn't agree at all. Inside, I screamed "No!"

But I was the youngest, the only girl, and there were three of them saying this is the right thing to do. I didn't stand a chance, so I kept quiet, nodding my head in agreement, but my world shattered at that moment. My heart broke even before I understood the immensity of that decision. And it would continue to break over and over for many years.

On that day, the belief that others get to interpret how I feel was planted deep within me. For the "family decision", I went along with mom and my brothers because I didn't know how to do anything else. In my position in the family, which held a human equivalent to "a pecking order" among animals, I was the youngest and the weakest, and so my wishes didn't matter. My mother and my brothers outnumbered me and overpowered me, and they got to tell me what to feel, because they were bigger, older, and stronger than I. That's what I learned as the youngest in the shadow of two older brothers. And I stayed in that shadow where I remained a victim long after I was out of their reach.

The trips to the farm stopped, along with the delicious noon meals at the wooden table. After my parents divorced, we were no longer welcome. My sense of security melted away like the butter on my mashed potatoes.

THREE:

Dirt poor

My mom was a divorced woman in the late '60s, at a time when it was not acceptable to be divorced. Society had strict rules of conduct, and being divorced essentially left a scarlet letter on a woman's chest. Women also faced inequality in terms of rights and pay, and often didn't receive enforcement for child support payments. At that time, my dad had another family to care for, so he chose not to pay my mom anything, ever, in support. And for making this choice, nothing happened to him. But a lot happened to us.

Later in life, when my mom could have taken his house and all he owned for a lifetime of back child support, she let bygones be bygones. I never understood why she forgave every cent he owed. My mom took the high road; she forgave him- which to this day, I don't get. The forgiveness, I get. But allowing him to get away with abandonment, skirting his financial and moral responsibilities, seemed like her path to martyrdom.

We moved away from our small town to Grand Island, Nebraska, and lived in a rental house while my mom went out into the world to make a living. She had a high school diploma and had been a stay-at-home mom since she was 18. She took underpaid work as a secretary. I didn't realize how hard things were for her until years later. She was a woman alone, with three kids, and no child support, living and working in a man's world. She would go to work all day, come home exhausted, and fall asleep on the couch until our bedtime. It turns out she was anemic, and being the giving person she was, she gave her rare blood type away, draining her own body of the nutrients it needed.

Mom was often too tired to cook, so my oldest brother, Jeff, took on the role of feeding us. He made flat hamburger patties that were overcooked and under seasoned. He'd open up a can of baked beans and we'd eat them right out of the can. Instead of gathering around the table as a family, the three of us often ate off paper plates standing at the counter, covering the leather-like burgers with ketchup. Our fast food-like meals mirrored our new family status- tough, cheap, and tossed in the trash.

I don't know where Jeff learned to make fudge, but somewhere along the way, he did. What he didn't learn was how to share. I can still see the white porcelain plate, slathered with chocolaty goodness, butter knife cuts marking the portions. Half or more of the batch was for him, and the rest was to be split between me and my brother, Mike. Since my brothers were both older, I rarely got my share. Once held on my daddy's lap, spoon-fed like a princess, I was now pushed to the bottom of the pile, begging for scraps like a dog.

We paid dearly for my dad's lack of character. There was a time, we had only one light bulb in the house. My mom took bulbs out of sockets when the electricity bill was more than she could pay. At night, we would move the lone bulb from room to room and fight over who got to use it. Of course, being unsupervised for hours at a time led to many fights between my two brothers- and between them and me. I always lost until I learned not to fight at all. I learned instead to rollover and give up before you were pummeled or shunned- but begging was still on the table, and I learned to do that pretty well.

Our family survived, one month at a time. My mom was resourceful and never let us go hungry. There was a popular local restaurant where they sold buckets of discarded chicken parts out the back door for cheap. What most people threw away became our delicacies. My mom made the best fried chicken and could even make chicken backs and gizzards taste good. She used a paper bag, flour, and water to coat the pieces, and then fried them in Crisco. They were perfectly seasoned- crispy on the outside, tender on the inside. There isn't much meat on the back of a chicken, so we learned to clean the meat off of a bone like scavengers.

The restaurant also sold fifty-pound sacks of potatoes for next to nothing. Growing up, I ate a lot of potatoes- fried, boiled, broiled, mashed, and hashed. Fried potatoes were our favorite. Thin slices browned up fast in the pan. With salt and ketchup, their taste resembled French fries. The hash I hated (and still do), but frequently it was all we had, so you either ate it or you went hungry.

Cornflakes were the only cereal we had in the house for most of my childhood. They were cheap and they came in economy-sized boxes. When I was sitting on my dad's lap, they were the best thing I ever ate, but without him, they made me sick. They became soggy pieces of cardboard swimming around in my bowl and there wasn't enough sugar on the planet to make them taste like they once did. To this day, I can't eat hash or cornflakes. I'd go hungry before I would make myself eat either.

That time in our lives was about survival. My mom did what she had to do in order to keep a roof over our heads and food in our stomachs. I recall an occasional picnic in the park with fried chicken and potato salad, but shared meals around the table is not something I remember happening much. I know nothing went to waste.

We reused or recycled everything, and we learned to walk the ditches along the road, scrounging for glass pop bottles, which we turned in for nickels and dimes. I didn't realize we were poor, or why. Strolling through the ditches, looking for the gleam of a coke bottle nestled beneath waist-high grass was a fun pastime. And at the end of the rainbow was candy or a cream soda, bought with the change from the bottles we gathered along the way.

As hard as my mom tried, wolves still came to the door. They came in the stack of unpaid bills, notices to shut off the power, worn out clothes, shoes too small and empty cupboards. My mom never gave up. She worked long hours and deprived herself of essentials to provide for us. We always had just enough. There were no social services, Medicaid, or help programs for my mom. No child support enforcement, no wage garnishment ever came to our rescue.

So, when a handsome man she'd been dating proposed to her, she gladly accepted. Theirs was a short courtship, but long enough for the three of us to know that we liked the guy. He was kind, brought us gifts, and let us pick the name of his new dog.

FOUR:

Winning the lottery

Dwayne lived on a farm, was well over six feet tall, and had blonde hair and sideburns. To me, he was a giant of a man- not just in stature, but also in how he treated me. Life for us kids went from dire to the best place on earth.

The farmhouse Dwayne occupied as a bachelor was outdated, oversized, and filthy. Filled with stacks of boxes, debris, and endless clutter, it needed care, which was a project that my mom took on with gusto. She cleaned, painted, and remodeled the dead house, and it came alive under her hand, and so did we. I remember she had the dining room painted a deep blue. It was the most beautiful color I'd ever seen, and I always loved being in that room. White lace curtains framed the large windows, adding a feminine touch and contrast to the oak trim. There were a lot of good meals and fond memories served in that dining room. Each of us had an assigned seat at the table, and we ate together, family style.

Since my mom no longer had to work, she was free to be a wife and a mom.

I don't recall eating one chicken back or bowl of cornflakes on the farm. Eggs Benedict became one of my favorite meals. I think preparing it was a trick my mom used to get me to eat the plentiful supply of eggs on the farm, but I didn't care. As soon as she added creamy hollandaise sauce, Canadian bacon, and English muffins I never resisted eggs again. In fact, I begged for more, especially if I was sick. That meal symbolized a time when, once again, I felt loved and nurtured. I still missed my dad, but with Dwayne around and my mom home, it felt like we were a proper family. All the broken pieces inside of me fit back together again.

They don't make houses like that farmhouse anymore- strong and sturdy, with solid wood trim. Our new family felt like that farmhouse to me. The best part of the house for us kids was the upstairs. A wide wooden staircase with a matching banister led the way to our haven. We each had our own room, with large windows looking out at the farm. There was plenty of room to play both inside and out of the house, with endless areas to explore and roam upon and be free. Hide and seek took on a whole new meaning and became our favorite game. You could hide for hours before the looker found you, especially if we played outside.

Dwayne, or D.R. as everyone called him, let us ride in the combine cab when harvest time came. He played his music loud to drown out the sound of the machine devouring the corn as we plugged along. Watching the sea of yellow pour into the back of the truck was entertaining too. My dad always seemed to get irritated when the three of us kids were around. In contrast, D.R. found new ways to include or entertain us.

He was friendly, outgoing, and talked a lot. I didn't care if he talked all the time, because he let me traipse along behind him, helping do chores and asking endless questions. He'd carry two five-gallon buckets to water or feed the animals. I was not only young and impressionable, but also small for my age, so watching him carry those buckets, slinging them around like they were weightless, impressed me a great deal. I couldn't imagine how anyone could be that strong. I was in awe of this giant of a man.

"How do you carry all that?" I'd ask, wide-eyed. "Isn't that heavy?"

"What's that for?"

"Why do you do that?"

I must have driven him crazy with my questions, but he rarely showed irritation. He'd lift me up on the side of the feed trough so I could watch him pour the feed as the cattle pushed and shoved their way towards the choicest morsels. It was always a fresh adventure following him around, and I never tired of the daily chores. Every day was fresh for me, like a present to open, not knowing what it contained but being delighted to find something new waiting within it for me. I'd ooh and aah at almost everything.

My brothers had it good, too. Dwayne bought them a minibike (small motorcycle) on which they could tear around the farm. For two adventurous boys, the farm was a piece of heaven. A farm is not only fun, but wrought with danger, and we did our fair share of living on the edge. I'm not sure our mom knew half of what Dwayne let us do, but it sure was fun!

We rode inside giant tractor tire rims, bracing ourselves against the sides as D.R. drove slowly along. Climbing the giant mound of harvested corn in the metal storage building kept us entertained for hours. We'd be waist deep in the corn, scrambling our way to the top as a wave of kernels slid down toward the auger. It was a game you had to be careful playing, and D.R. was there, yelling at us to stay out of the way. We laughed and relished in our freedom but we were ever conscious of the danger we flirted with. Sliding into a spinning auger would be mutilation or death.

Riding atop corn in the back of a red wood-sided truck, lying flat against the pile of kernels was a favorite experience. The only thing more fun than that was riding home in the empty truck after they had weighed the corn. Once the truck bed was bare, a new game started. Giant chains hung above from one side of the wood slat walls to the other. They held the sides together as the weight of corn pushed against them. There were three chains spaced evenly apart overhead- one for each of us. A layer of grain dust covered the bed floor and turned it into a skating rink. The three of us would grab a chain and swing and slide recklessly back and forth as D.R. drove the truck home.

Abandoned wood buildings were for exploring, and for hiding in, but you had to be careful of wasp nests. Chickens roamed free during the day and were great fun to chase, until the rooster came after you. On our farm, there were farm cats with kittens to cuddle, along with several dogs, and sometimes a batch of puppies.

Our family story turned from tragedy to "You won the lottery." I was the happiest I had ever been as a child. Life on a farm suited us, and opened a new world of endless fun.

And it got even better one Christmas. In my mind, the only thing missing in this utopia was a horse, and I never stopped asking for one. With acres of pasture, I knew there was room for one. Money didn't seem to be an issue, and we had more than enough food to eat, so when Christmas rolled around, it was all I could talk about. I still believed in Santa Claus, and I was sure that he would bring me a horse that year. My family teased me, telling me every reason Santa could not bring me a horse. But my child's heart shut them all out. I knew there would be a horse.

The drive home from the Christmas Eve church service seemed to take forever. My heart raced as we drove the dirt roads back to the farm. As the headlights turned into our driveway, the outline of a horse tied to the fence in our front yard caught my eye and I squealed with excitement. It's a good thing Santa came through or I might have given up on life at the tender age of eight.

Under the Christmas tree was a bridle, a halter, lead rope, and brushes. Peace and goodwill came into our lives, and we won the lottery on a little farm in Nebraska, with a man named Dwayne.

FIVE:

Too good to be true

Life has taught me that if something seems too good to be true, it probably is. There is no paradise on earth, especially in small town Nebraska. Life seemed idyllic, and I'm sure my brothers felt the same way. D.R. was good to us, and it was obvious he adored our mom. He showered her with gifts, indulged her every wish, and expressed his love often- so what could go wrong?

The first sign of trouble showed up one day on our doorstep. I found D.R. lying face down on the cement. Vomit spewed around him. He was sick! I ran to tell my mom. Her reaction was not what I expected. She didn't seem to care. My mom was a caregiver extraordinaire, so I was confused. Whenever we were sick, my mom took excellent care of us, fussing and fretting until we were well again- so why didn't she rush to help Dwayne?

Slurred speech, unsteady gait, and passing out in your own vomit might have been telltale signs for an adult, but as a child, it confused me. It was years later before I understood the problem. Dwayne would do anything for my mom, except stay sober. And by the time he got sober, it was too late.

I think life likes to be cruel, because what happened next shattered our world and left us homeless. Our second Christmas Eve together turned out much differently than the one we shared the year before. That night we drove the same dirt road to and from church, anticipating a fun-filled Christmas on the farm. What greeted us at home were crimson flames glowing from the front window of our newly remodeled farmhouse.

Fire is like a living beast. It's ferocious, and it takes what it wants. It does not stop until it consumes everything in its path and leaves behind the putrid stench of death. Black death. Everything remaining is covered in ash and soot, destroyed beyond recognition.

You can't find your favorite Snoopy stuffed animal, despite days spent searching the blackened rubble. You have lost your family pictures and heirlooms forever. If any of your clothes are not charred, they will still smell so bad you will never wear them again.

"Merry Christmas- life as you know it is over." That's what the hungry beast screamed. Our lives then tumbled down like the remains of that house. Where happiness and beauty once stood, destruction took hold and chipped away at the fragile structure of our lives.

The first to go was our home. Next came a harsh realization that the foundation of my mom's marriage was a lie. D.R. had posed as a knight in shining armor, and my mom, the damsel in distress. They each had played their part perfectly. Her distress was real; his chivalry, not so much. He was all but bankrupt, with bills and loans looming large. And he was an alcoholic. One minute he was the life of the party, and the next, he was a blackout drunk. His condition left mom alone to deal with the fire aftermath, and to fight with the insurance agent about a claim from our makeshift home, a trailer house pulled onto the property. And fight she did.

On one of the insurance adjuster's visits, I saw her rise to the challenge. I had a pet mouse that somehow survived the fire. My room was located upstairs on the opposite side of where the fire had started, so smoke only damaged that corner of the house. Whiskers, my pet white mouse with pink-rimmed eyes, had survived unscathed. I kept him in a glass aquarium with sawdust shavings on the bottom and a wire mesh top. Mice are tiny Houdini's in disguise. They can jump high and squeeze through openings much smaller than their bodies. All it takes is one lapse of security (like forgetting to place the brick atop the wire mesh) and that mouse is running free.

"Mom, umm, something bad happened," I said, right before the insurance man arrived.

"Like, what?" my mom asked.

"Whiskers. I can't find him."

A knock on the front door came just in time to save me. The insurance adjuster entered our humble space. I don't recall the words used, but it was clear he didn't want to pay us enough money for our claim. My mom was mad. I sensed she hated this man and if my mom didn't like him, he must be terrible because my mom was nice to everyone.

He sat at the table, across from my mom, as they glared at one another. Gone was the solid wood table and the beautiful blue walls. My mom no longer cared who sat where for meals because there wasn't enough room for all of us in this room, anyways. The spacious kitchen she once enjoyed was a memory. Now she had a barbie-doll sink with two feet of counter space, and a card table with wobbly legs where we ate meals, and by which she and the adjuster sat.

In Nebraska, when tragedy strikes, neighbors bring mounds of food. Our tiny fridge and counters were stacked with home-made pies, casseroles, and freshly baked bread. But I don't recall eating any of it. Food was abundant, but our lives were empty and the last thing I wanted was to eat. When your heart is broken, your stomach feels sick, at least mine did. The tipsy table seemed appropriate for our circumstances. No matter how many home-cooked meals our friends brought, it felt like we would, like that card table, collapse at any minute.

Nobody saw the white dot streak across the floor but me. I held my breath as Whiskers ran under the table. The insurance man stopped in mid-sentence, looking down at his right leg.

"What's that?" he asked, shaking his leg.

"What?" my mom asked.

"It feels like something just crawled up my leg."

"Hopefully it's a mouse," my mom said with a smile.

"A what?"

"My daughter's pet mouse went missing right before you arrived," she said.

The man's eyes widened as he stamped his foot and screamed like a baby, circling and stomping, trying to get Whiskers off his leg.

"Don't you dare hurt that mouse," my mom said through gritted teeth.

A streak of white hit the floor, and I scrambled after Whiskers. I dove under the table, cornering the frightened rodent against the wall, and scooped him up in my hands.

I always wondered if that mouse of a man peed his pants, because he left abruptly and slammed the door. Despite the shock waves that rocked the trailer, that flimsy card table held up. But soon, our family crumbled beneath the weight of everything upon us.

SIX:

Darkness enters

It wasn't long after the fire that Mom moved us off the farm into a trailer park on the edge of town. I assume D.R. continued to live in the trailer on the farm, but I never knew. Then, I was a walking zombie, still in shock over the fire, the move, and our losses. No details come to mind of saying goodbye to my horse, D.R., or the other animals, but I recall how awful I felt inside and didn't know what to do with those feelings. Dark clouds of depression followed me around like Charles Schulz's character, Pig-Pen, in the Peanuts comic strip.

It would be hard as an adult to manage the tragedy, and the subsequent divorce, but it is much harder for a child. That's where and when my depression began, and it was the seedbed for my future eating disorders. I locked the pain I felt so deep in my soul that it became a permanent part of me. I'm sure we talked about these painful things as a family, but I don't remember any discussions.

When my dad left us, I was sad, but going through this ca-
tastrophe was, for me, an emotional death. It was worse than
eating chicken backs or fighting over a lone light bulb because, at least during that period, I was fighting to live. Now,
my body was limp and felt heavy, like a dead corpse, as I
dragged it around.

The four walls of our trailer house closed tight around me.
I longed for my spacious bedroom looking out on the farm.
Now, I couldn't breathe in this mobile home. The air within
was heavy, and the old rented trailer smelled foul. Used to
having an entire farm to roam, I felt bored out of my mind in
our new home, and yet too tired to care. Depression drained
my energy or desire to do anything. I sat in the back of the
trailer, throwing a ball against a cardboard wall between my
propped-up feet. Thwap, pause. Thwap, pause.

By now, there were no tears. I was beyond feeling. This was
the abyss I had silently slipped into- a world devoid of light,
because to feel was too much for me.

Injustice! My heart screamed. How could I be so happy one
day and end up so miserable the next? We went from living in
Disneyland to hell in one night. And it wasn't fair. *Hadn't we
suffered enough?*

My brothers were miserable, too, and soon directed their pain
toward me. A trailer house with three rambunctious kids soon
became cramped as tempers grew short.

I had long been the object of ridicule for my brothers, and a punching bag for them, but now there was no dad to teach them differently, or to stop them from being abusive, so their rage was turned on me. Mom was once again working long hours, which left us alone, and my brothers' behaviors unchecked, and her exhausted most of the time.

My Uncle Bill, my mother's younger brother, once witnessed my brothers' unacceptable behavior while staying with us on the farm and promptly put a stop to their abuse. He caught my brothers hitting me, and he turned the tables on them.

I'm sure if Dwayne or my mom had witnessed how rough my brothers were on me, they would have stopped their abuse, but my brothers were smart enough to beat up on me when Dwayne or my mom weren't around. And there was an unspoken pact between the three of us kids that I kept my mouth shut, no matter what they did to me, because if I tattled, we would all get spanked, and then, after they received their punishment, my brothers would make my life even harder. So, I learned to stay quiet and not tell my mom.

Mom and D.R. left my uncle in charge of us on many occasions while they went out, and some of my fondest memories are of the fun times we had while Uncle Bill was babysitting. As soon as Mom and D.R. walked out the door, we would turn over every piece of furniture and construct tent tunnels with blankets, sheets, and towels draped across the upturned furniture. We'd turn out all the lights and use flashlights to scurry through the labyrinth from one end to the other. Uncle Bill would watch the time and make sure we put everything back in its rightful place before Mom and D.R. returned. Part of the fun was the secrecy between us, getting away with something the adults didn't know about.

My brothers didn't guard their behavior toward me around Uncle Bill, since it felt like he was one of us. Ten years younger than my mother, Bill wasn't that much older than we were. Once, he caught them hitting me and warned them to stop or he would do the same to them. The next time he caught them, there was no warning, and he roughed them both up pretty good.

"How do you like it?" he asked. "Hurts, huh?" he asked as he pummeled them repeatedly.

Then he warned, "If you ever touch her again, I will beat you to a pulp. Never, ever hit a girl."

I remember very few times when I received justice, but that one instance made me feel good. It stopped the physical abuse for a long time, but by then, much damage to my spirit had already been done. The message to me was loud and clear. Take the abuse and don't complain or talk about it, and never, ever tattle.

Inevitably, Uncle Bill wasn't regularly around to make good on his threats, so in time, the pummeling began again. The beatings I took were nothing compared to the pain in my heart. Bruises on the outside heal, but bruises on the inside can last a lifetime.

SEVEN:

Hope springs

Life in a trailer park with a bicycle were not enough to keep us entertained, and I'm certain we pushed my mom to the edge of insanity, but she was ambitious with an indomitable spirit, so when she saw an opportunity to return us to farm life, she took it.

Our great-great-grandparents immigrated from Germany decades earlier and homesteaded land in Nebraska, where they lived and worked on the land, and had built a house, a barn, and several sheds. In time, my great-grandfather died while constructing a barn on the land, leading my great-grandmother to move to town and abandon the farm. My grandmother owned it after they passed, and as an only child, was its sole proprietor. My mom, with the help of my Uncle Bill, secured the use of the abandoned homestead from my grandmother, and they went into the hog business together.

The house my great-grandparents had lived in was long abandoned, and had no indoor plumbing. It was too small for our
family, and would have been costly to update for our needs, so
it remained empty. My mom solved the problem of where we
would live by bringing in a brand-new trailer house. This was
the 1970s, so red shag carpet adorned the floors, inviting us to
make ourselves at home. The trailer house was a far cry from
the spacious house we shared with D.R., but it sure beat living
in a smelly trailer park in town.

We spent months repairing the sheds worth saving, and tore
apart or burned down buildings too dilapidated to repair. Since
my uncle was a carpenter by trade, he built a farrowing house
where the pigs would give birth. I remember watching him
work, pouring the foundation, raising the trusses, and bringing
life back to the dead farm. Our spirits rose with every truss
that was put into place. Hope returned as we worked together,
painting all the buildings white with black trim except for the
enormous barn that my grandfather had built, and died for. It
remained a faded red, reminding us of the past and the sacrifice he made building it.

Blood, sweat, and tears went into the farm. We cleared brush,
chopped overgrown weeds and, together, created our future. It
would serve as a base for where the three of us kids could grow
up. We were back on a farm, and with my Uncle Bill there, it
felt like we were a family again.

My brothers left me alone while my uncle was around. They knew he would not hesitate to return any wrath they took out on me. I felt safe for the first time in months. Not having to look over my shoulder helped chase away the dark cloud following me around. The sun came up in my soul, especially when D.R. showed up again.

One day, he pulled up in a truck and trailer and in the back was the second greatest surprise of my life. Tied to the rail was a white and brown spotted pony (Appaloosa) and I knew he was mine! What I didn't understand was the argument that broke out between my mom and D.R. Something about the wrong horse. What was this, she asked?

This was Patches. My small hands clung to sides of the truck, trembling as I peeked at the pretty pony. He looked at me, eyes wide, and neighed.

"It's ok. I won't hurt you," I whispered. "We are going to be friends."

My mom didn't realize that what she thought was a mistake would be the greatest gift I ever received. Patches was a Welsh pony cross, smaller than most horses but bigger than most ponies. At 13.5 hands high, he was the perfect size. I'm convinced God himself chose that pony for me and sent him to save me. He was even-tempered, full of spunk, and smart. Patches taught me lessons that have lasted a lifetime and he was the best friend I ever had.

I rode Patches every chance I got. Across the road from our farm was an area we called the sand pit. There were steep hills and deep ditches covered in sand, which was the perfect place to learn to ride a rambunctious pony that tries to lose its rider. Patches was clever and lazy, so he devised new ways daily to dump me. I can't say I blame him, since I never tired of riding. There were pastures to explore, cornfields to cross, and endless roads to follow.

Patches was kid-proof. He didn't kick, bite, or buck. I taught him to let me stand upright on his back while he stood still, to let me leap on him from behind, and to ride backwards at a gallop. But when he got tired, he'd stop and lie down, right in the middle of the road or the trail. Saddle and all, he'd plop down and roll, trying to lose me and the contraption strapped to his back. Or if we were galloping along, he'd come to a sudden stop, lowering his head as I flew over it. If there was an open cornfield, he'd swerve down a row as the leaves blinded me and sliced my face and arms. Yep, Patches taught me how to stick to a horse, how to fall without breaking a bone, and to be ready for anything. He was the perfect companion for a young, adventurous girl.

When I was with my horse, the world was far away. The pain from divorce, fire, or fear of my brothers didn't exist. I was whoever I wanted to be. This was my fantasy realm, and my mind galloped away when I was riding.

Having a horse was much more than just riding to escape. It was a close connection to an animal that saved my soul. I could talk to Patches and tell him about my troubles. He'd perk his ears, and I knew he was listening. My secrets, my hopes, my fears were all safe with him. He could keep secrets better than anyone.

I felt one with my horse. When he galloped, I could feel his muscles ripple beneath as I followed the rhythm of each stride. If he twitched to flick a fly from his belly, I felt it in my legs. I spent hours riding bareback, and it taught me to feel my horse and expect what he would do next. If he tightened in fear, I knew before he bolted. Our connection went beyond words, into a spiritual realm. And that bond healed parts I never knew were broken.

Even though D.R. brought the pony, I knew it was my mom that arranged it. I will forever be grateful that she made sure I had a horse while growing up. She was a horse lover also, and understood that I not only wanted a horse, my soul *needed* a horse. I was a free spirit, prone to wander, preferred getting dirty to dressing up, and happiest outside with the animals. My brothers never took to horses, so I was free from them whenever I took off on Patches. My mind soared to new heights while astride my sturdy steed.

So much time spent with my horse allowed for hours of silence, and for me to be lost in my thoughts. It's where my creativity bloomed, and daydreaming became my favorite pastime. I'd create elaborate stories in my head, with dialog, plots, and conversations between characters. If I wasn't riding my horse, I was reading about riding or stories about animals, particularly dogs. I devoured every book I could get my hands on with those themes. Books were my escape, my inspiration, my friends.

And that is when I realized that I differed from other kids my age- not that other kids didn't read or daydream, but- because I made up stories and played them out in my head. Elaborate scenarios of faraway places, interesting characters, and conversations held between them would pop into my brain and take over my thoughts.

I would pretend to be those people, changing my voice to match the character, having hours of fun imagining what they might say or do. It was something I could not stop. It just happened, particularly when I was outside. And I didn't have to be alone. If I was in a lull, my mind would go somewhere else and create a new story. At age ten, I put pen to paper and wrote my first book, titled Cowboy the Wild Mustang.

I knew it was weird that my mind took me to where it wanted to go, so I never spoke of it or told anyone about it, because how could they possibly understand it when I didn't? As a child, I didn't realize it was a gift, or know what to do with it. I'm sure it was an escape mechanism my mind had developed to deal with the pain and challenges I'd experienced. I now see it for what it is, a vivid imagination and the burning desire to be a writer.

There is always a story inside of me waiting to come out. When other writers speak of being blocked, I smile, because I have so many stories going on at one time, I could never write them all. Even at sixty, my imagination runs wild like I am ten again. It is to be celebrated and I no longer fear that I'm going crazy. I channel it to weave stories and eventually books.

Something happens when I'm out in nature. Perhaps it's the energy that the earth, trees, and plants emit that fuel my creativity. I don't know, and I no longer care what others think. I just know it works and if I need to get inspired, I go for a hike. You see two telephone poles on a hill with a dirt path. I see a dragon castle with a gold road leading through a drawbridge. I work out plots, dialog, and create characters, both good and bad, for my stories while walking along, often talking to myself.

There were several years of relative peace in our home on our farm. Hard work drains excess energy that might otherwise be directed negatively toward others. But at that time, my uncle was young and restless. He had his own dragons to slay, princesses to rescue, and wild seeds to sow. And so, eventually, he left us and went off to seek his fortune. I was young and didn't know what happened for sure, or why he and my mom ended their partnership. But without his brawn and the balance he brought, the kingdom crumbled piece by piece and, again, our world fell apart.

EIGHT:

Reality sucks

When Uncle Bill left, there was no longer an alpha male around, and my protective shield went with him. Now, my brothers were older, stronger, and full of hormones. It was not a wonderful combination for me or for them.

Teenage boys left without a leader will take over, and among us siblings, my oldest brother Jeff became the boss. Firstborn, he was a natural leader, but he lacked the maturity of a man, and thrust into a role beyond his years, he stepped up, stepped on, and stepped over all of us. Jeff was intelligent, driven, and had the Midas touch, and to me, he was the golden child. He was good looking, athletic, and well-liked at school. At home, he was a bit of a bully.

One time, he brought home a frozen pizza for himself and cooked it in front of me as I begged for a piece. He tired of my pleading and forced me to eat the entire pizza by myself. I was four years his younger, small for my age, and a girl. What was easy for a teenage boy with a bottomless pit to consume was torment for me to finish. Through tears, I begged him to let me stop eating, but he would not let me leave until every bite was gone. By the time I began the last piece, I gagged at the smell of pepperoni. My stomach was now stretched past capacity and every bite became torture. Tears streamed down my face as the hard, dry crust choked me going down. I regretted begging for a piece, swearing to myself that I would never again ask him for anything. The only lesson I learned that day was that food was a control weapon to use against someone.

Jeff didn't bully just me. He was an equal opportunity kind of guy and shared the fun with my other brother, Mike. We were each two years apart, and Mike was the middle child. Jeff and Mike had a complicated relationship that I never understood. They were best buddies one minute, and trying to kill each other the next. Jeff would goad Mike and tease him until he lost his temper, often by cheating at ping-pong and then claiming victory.

Jeff was a bully, but Mike was dangerous when he got mad. There was a time they argued and Mike grabbed a baseball bat. Jeff locked himself in the bathroom and stayed there until Mom came home.

"What ya doing?" Mom asked, seeing Mike sitting on the floor, leaning against the locked bathroom door.

"Waiting," Mike said.

"For what?" asked Mom.

"For Jeff to come out," Mike said, holding the bat in one hand, and tapping the other with it.

Good thing, Jeff, made it to the bathroom in time.

As Jeff got older, he stopped pummeling me, but Mike long took his rage out on me with his fists. I learned three major lessons from Mike: how to take a beating, what anguish is, and how to make myself throw up.

My revenge for Mike was not to cry when he beat on me. I'd turn and stand there until he finished pounding out his rage on my back. A steel reserve kept me from crying. He liked to see tears and hear me sob, so not expressing the pain he inflicted upon me became my weapon.

One day, my tactic backfired though, as he became enraged when he couldn't get the reaction he wanted from me, and he turned to attack a vulnerable spot in me. Creative by nature, I loved to draw and paint. I was proud of my work, especially since it was a talent my brothers did not possess. They were dominant in many things, but making art, that was my gift. That day, Mike grabbed and busted my prized creation over his knee- a white bunny rabbit with a baby-blue background I'd painted on a piece of wood. My heart shattered along with the artwork as I cried.

That experience was the first time I understood anguish. Much different from pain or grief, anguish comes with having a broken heart and spirit, where the pain you feel is so deep you fall to your knees, unable to breathe, and wail. That is anguish. It is the activation of years of accumulated hurt, set off through one violent act.

No justice came to Mike that day, or any day, for his offenses. There was no one to step in and make him pay for his sins. If my mom was around, she did nothing to him. The lack of justice I felt that day when he destroyed my prized possession took my soul and set me up for what was to become my battlefield.

My brothers often treated me as an inconvenience and a source of amusement.

In the winter, they would use me to scout saucer sled routes down steep slopes at the sandpit. To see if a fresh path was safe, they would make me go down it first. I'd scream, cry, and beg as they released the round coaster of death, sending me forth, regardless of my pleas. It must have been great fun for them to watch me fly down a steep, snow-covered hill in the sandpit, screaming in fear. Despite the craziness, I continued to follow along with them and learned to avoid complaining, or they would leave me behind. Little sisters want to be part of the action. My fear of missing out and wanting to belong with them was greater than my fear of getting hurt. I was as sick as they were.

There was one particularly cruel game they played with me without my permission, and I would have opted out of it if I could. They placed a pillow over my face while they tickled me until I peed my pants. A deep-seated fear of not being able to breathe and a hatred of being tickled remains to this day. I won't attempt to dive underwater- ever- because I'm fearful of not being able to breathe. Even learning to snorkel years later was difficult for me because every time the water hit my face, I freaked out.

Where was my mom when these things were happening? I don't know. Outside, working with the pigs, or asleep on the couch, hiding from the world, is what little I remember of her presence in those day. What I do know is that the weight of the world was on her shoulders and, at some point, she sought her own solace. I recall bottles of bourbon- big ones- stuck under the kitchen cupboard, and under the back seat of her car that rolled out when we stopped. Even now, the smell of bourbon makes me sick to my stomach. Though I don't recall her drinking it, one whiff of the nasty stuff wrinkles my nose and makes me turn away.

At that age, I was too young to know that I was at risk. All I remember was riding with her in the car, ecstatic when we would stop somewhere along the way. She would get one of those adult beverages in a can and I would get candy or a soda. To me, it was fun to go places with her because the stops were frequent and I got a reward each time.

Until she went away.

My Aunt Gloria sat on the stairs outside of our trailer house, trying to explain why I was coming to stay with her for the summer. My mom was sick and had to go to a place where she could get better. The stress of being a single mom, the responsibilities of the farm, and the pain left over from the divorce must have been too much for her, and my mom suffered a nervous breakdown. I did not know what that was, but I was to experience it myself years later.

The signs were there, but as a child, I wasn't aware of what was happening with her. She slept a lot, but she was always tired. She overate, often bingeing, and she became obese, spending most of her time on the couch.

Our new trailer house became a cluttered mess with dirty dishes and debris stacked high about it, while overgrown weeds took over our yard. I imagine that there were a lot of unpaid bills in the piles of papers here and there. When we were younger, she took great pride in our home and often sang along with her favorite records as she cleaned the house. But stress, depression, and anxiety had robbed her of life. At this time, she turned to food and the bottle to cope until even those didn't relieve the emotional pressure she was feeling. Our family now looked like the trailer trash we were, and it was during this time that my own unhealthy eating habits formed.

My mom and I set up battle lines for control early on. By forcing me to eat what I didn't like, meal times became a game between her will and mine. She could make me do a lot of things, but eating wasn't one of them. No threat, punishment, or hours forced to sit alone at the table could make me eat if I didn't want to. Going to bed hungry wasn't enough to make me lose my grip on the only control I had in this dysfunctional family. And I later learned to use it against her and flip the finger at the world.

However, the pendulum swung the other way for me as I got older, when an abundance of food on the farm made it easy to go from being forced to eat to runaway bingeing.

The freezer was always full with bacon, ham, and pork chops. Eating fried foods was our norm, and since sugar and flour were cheap, they became our staples. Jiffy cake, cornbread, and muffin mixes were popular then, as well, as they were the first prepared baking mixes on the market- and they were easy enough for me to make. Just add water and an egg to the mix, and bake. Blueberry muffins and chocolate cake were my personal favorites, so I made them often. I slathered sickeningly sweet canned frosting on top of cakes. Once I learned how to make chocolate chip cookies from scratch, life was never the same.

NINE:

Perfection

At twelve, my idea of perfection appeared. Her name was Carmen. She was everything I was not, and it was clear the boys thought she was perfect, too, because she got asked to the dance on the last night of Bible camp and I didn't.

If I was a boy, I'd have asked her too. She had blue eyes, straight blonde hair that fell to the middle of her back, high cheekbones, long arms and legs, and no cellulite. The classic American beauty in my world.

Had I grown up in a different time, place, or culture, I might not have been so hard on myself. Here in New Mexico, where I now live, girls with dark hair and ample curves are an ideal of beauty, both in American Indian and Spanish-speaking circles. They are voluptuous, and are proud of it. Where I came from, if you had a spare tire, ample bosom or a bouncy butt, you tried to cover it up or hide it, and not let it spill over with pride.

In these New Mexico communities, they celebrate themselves, their people, and their cultures- what they are- with elaborate feasts, ceremonies, and music. Bright colors adorn bodies and are used to decorate doors, fences, homes and jewelry.

My dark, curly hair might have been normal in one of these cultures, and perhaps I would have grown it long and relished in it, but in a small town in Nebraska, it was a curse. Heat, humidity, and ignorance added to my humility. No one knew what to do with my crazy curls. If you combed or brushed it, it frizzed more, and blow drying it demolished it. So, we cut it short and kept it short. That was cute when I was young, but as I got older and chubbier, my hair got bigger. Fluffy, that's what it was. Big and fluffy. Like a ball of fuzz on top of my head. Not what any teenage girl wanted. If I had a dollar for every time people asked me if my hair was real, I'd be rich by now.

"Is your hair real?"

"Yes. Why would I do this to myself?" That is the answer I wanted to give them.

Instead, I'd smile and say "Yes."

Most men prefer long hair, and I spent a good portion of my life trying to please them, wishing for Carmen-like locks. But my curls make me unique, like an icon. My hair is as stubborn as I am and refuses to follow the crowd. It will do as it chooses and you can't make it behave- any more than someone could make me eat when I was in the depth of my eating disorder.

I still think about Carmen. I wonder what she looks like now. Would I still wish I looked like her? Did she age well? Probably not, I think to myself, and smile.

Perfection. That was the goal. To be anything less than perfect was to be unacceptable. Unlovable. That's the belief that I carried in my head. It's also the concept that led me down the dark path of doom. Perfection existed only in my mind, but I didn't realize it until years later. It was the driving force behind everything I did.

Who decides what or who is perfect? Is there a "Perfection Committee" out there, casting votes for or against us? If there was such a thing, I suspect they would have been much easier on me than I was on myself. We are our own worst critics, and for someone with an eating disorder- particularly anorexia- harsh judgment becomes the norm until the standards get twisted into unrealistic expectations.

Magazine, billboard and television ads shove idealism down our throats. They send us the message that successful people are thin and beautiful. For most models, the thinner you are, the better. They parade young, often pubescent girls with bony shoulders, stringy legs, and little to no muscularity as the ideal. I can't imagine the pressure those girls feel. It is great if you are born with it, but torture if you are the average American girl or boy. I knew a model who said that in order to stay svelte, she only ate a few times a week. On the other days, she fasted, consuming only water. When I suggested that maybe this wasn't a healthy lifestyle, she became defensive and reminded me that fasting is good for our bodies. Sure, once in a while, but not as a lifestyle.

Skaters, gymnasts, ballerinas, and dancers are among those expected to maintain slim physiques. Pressure to fit into a mold created by our society can lead to a lifelong eating disorder or worse.

But where did my pursuit of perfectionism come from? My mother never expected perfection. She told me often that I could be anything I wanted, that I was special, and that she was proud of me, so it wasn't her doing. My dad told me he loved me, but his actions spoke louder than his words.

As our family struggled to make ends meet, his family lived in a big two-story house and had what seemed to me like everything. Especially my stepsister. She was part of the package that my dad inherited. Several years older and a couple inches taller than me, I might have looked up to her had she not been such a spoiled brat. As an only child until her baby brother came along, she was used to getting her way. My mom sent us to stay with my dad and his new family for several weeks one summer. I'm sure his wife never dreamed she'd be stuck with the three of us for any length of time. It was clear when we arrived that her daughter didn't plan on accommodating us either.

She could scream louder and longer than anyone I ever met. Hurling hate, kicking, and using expletives that weren't allowed in our home, she spat vile names at her mother and towards us. I didn't know how to handle such behavior, especially when she directed it towards me. She bossed me around and used her size to torment me. Once again, I was the underdog.

My mouth dropped open the first time I entered her room. There, before a closet bursting with clothes, and beneath white lace curtains, a matching bedspread and skirt wrapped around a white, four-poster bed frame which sat on pink shag carpet. The scene was complete with a Barbie Dreamhouse with the matching pink corvette. I was in awe of all her things and couldn't believe their family lived like kings while we suffered as paupers. You would think a girl that lived in that room would be as sweet as her surroundings, but I soon discovered just how wicked a stepsister could be. It was clear who ran the house, and it wasn't my dad.

When no one was looking, she'd push me around, jab an elbow in my ribs and stick her tongue out at me, and then smile as though nothing had ever happened. I was used to being bullied by my brothers, but this felt worse. My brothers made their dominance known to her early on, so she left them alone, except to scream at the top of her lungs for her mom if they even got close to her. Together, she and I might have had a chance against the boys, but she preferred to throw tantrums over combining forces. Unless she wanted to play Barbies. Then, I was her best friend. Her on-and-off thing confused me. In my world, either you liked someone, or you didn't- and if you didn't, the last thing you did was to invite them into your room to play.

This was the closest I ever got to having a sister. It was also my first introduction into the world of girldom. I was used to boys and their rough and tumble ways. This world was foreign to me, but inside, I enjoyed playing dress-up, having tea parties and playing with Barbies. We would shut the boys out of her room and play together for hours on the pink floor. I'm not sure what they were up to while we dressed our Barbie and Ken dolls in the latest fashions, but I didn't care. For once, I got to play pretend with someone other than my horse. And it was fun until she got bossy.

"Give me that one. She's mine. Here, you can have this one," she said, as she thrust the old Barbie doll my way.

The doll's head barely stayed on her plastic neck, and she had dark hair with a choppy cut. My stepsister always got the blonde with big boobs and shiny hair.

"Don't do it that way. Here, let me show you how to dress her properly," as she yanked the Barbie back.

I'd sit there, unsure of what to do. I was compliant most of the time. Until one day she pushed me too far.

It wasn't jealousy over things that caused me to explode that day. I was never comfortable in her world and didn't wish that I lived in her house. I never wanted to be like her, because she was so unlikeable. It wasn't the material things they had that bothered me, but *who* they had taken from us that seemed so unfair. The baby was helpless and not to blame. It wasn't his fault. He was the product of my selfish father and my stepsister's careless mother. It was much later that I understood all of this, but I understood one thing clearly at that time.

My stepsister had my dad and demanded his attention, and yet she didn't want him. The man I loved with my whole heart she treated like crap. And because of her mom, my dad let her. All my stepsister wanted were the things that he could give her. All I wanted was his love, but he gave what little he had to them.

Those feelings came pouring out that day when I hit her.

We were outside, taking turns riding her bicycle. It was pink, of course, with a white banana seat, white grips with the plastic strings hanging down, and a white wicker basket on the front, mounted between the handlebars. A pink bike wouldn't have been my first choice, but it was the only entertainment we had for outside fun. It was my turn to ride, but she grabbed the bike away from me and the handle bar clipped me on the chin. And it hurt. I remember looking down at my doubled-up fist, right before it connected with her face. It felt like an out-of-body experience, as though I was watching someone else hit my stepsister. For the first time in my young life, I fought back. And won.

She dropped the bike, ran towards the house screaming for her mommy, and I got to ride alone- until she raised the rafters with her threats. I looked up at her, glaring down from her second-story room as she yelled through the glass.

"I'm going to kill you!"

"I hate you!"

"Just wait until I get my hands on you!"

My heart pounded. I hadn't thought of the consequences of my actions. She was bigger than I and could beat me to a pulp. I ran to my brothers for protection, begging them to help me.

They asked nonchalantly what happened. It must have been funny to them because they smiled. Their little sister hit the big bully.

I think they would have protected me if it came down to me versus her. I will never know for sure, because they never had to. Her threats were empty. She never bullied me again. I learned an important lesson that day: if you stand up to a bully, they will probably run. On the outside, they are all show, but on the inside is a big baby. Especially in her case, when she was outnumbered, three to one.

My stepmother kept her house pristine. I swear nothing was ever out of place, especially in the sitting room, furnished in white. The sofa and the chairs stood like ghosts on a bed of bleached carpet. Long, luxurious drapes framed the windows, adding the finishing touch of class. She never allowed us in that room. My young mind didn't understand the purpose of such a space. Our trailer house could have fit into their combined living and dining room. It must have been expensive to support two cars, a big house, a new baby, and a spoiled brat. No wonder my dad didn't pay his child support. Every dime he made went to provide for this family.

My mom sent us with one change of clothes to force my dad into buying us new things. The few times he let me pick out items from the clothing store he owned, it flooded me with guilt. I was used to my mom sacrificing for us, but when my dad did something nice for us, I felt guilty about it. And I made a *big* deal over what he did, like it was the greatest thing in the world. As though I wasn't worth such things and I owed him a debt. My brothers and I lived in a world where, when one of us got new shoes, we oohed and aahed over them, happy for the recipient.

If I had the chance to speak to my younger self, I'd say, "Are you kidding? Look around, girl, at what they have and never feel bad about accepting anything from your dad again."

At their house, there was a fancy wood table in the dining room, and a small round table in the kitchen where we ate most of our meals. The only thing I remember eating was cinnamon and sugar toast. A white plastic container held the brown and white mixture. A small lid popped open on one side for sprinkling, while the other side had a wide lid for pouring in the ingredients. I was used to cheap grape jam piled on warm toast with butter, but this treat became my favorite. We'd remove the ugly green cover from the toaster, plug it in and wait for our warm piece of toast to pop up. Between the four of us kids, we could eat a lot of toast. I never liked the appliance covers- they seemed like a waste of time and money- but my stepmom must have loved them, because she had dotted her kitchen with the matching sewage-green colored appliance covers.

Every night after dinner, she'd load the dishwasher, wipe her hands on a kitchen towel, and cover up all the appliances, as though she was tucking them into bed. If I wandered through the kitchen at night, the awful green covers were there, hiding the mixer, the coffee pot and the toaster. I wondered how many times a day she had to put them on and pull them off. Nothing was out of place in that house, except my brothers and me. My stomach felt like the color of the dreaded covers when I stayed there. Everything was too perfect there- except me.

Poverty taught me to appreciate the smallest things- to find delight and contentment in simple pleasures- which is a lesson I'm not sure my stepsister and brother ever got, but one I am grateful to have learned. Their family lived like kings, while my dad had discarded our family like trailer trash. The picture before me then was clear: If I am perfect, my dad will love me.

TEN:

Transition
Adolescent years

My brothers were athletic and popular. I was forever in their shadows and never felt like I was good enough. I understood their peers only accepted me because I was the little sister. At least, that's what I thought.

Jeff was good at football, made an all-star team, and might have had a lucrative career had it not been for his inherited back problems. One wrong hit, the doctor said, could leave him paralyzed for life. Jeff quit football and turned his ambition to work, making and saving money like a madman until he had enough for a down payment on a brand-new black Trans Am. His popularity was unmatched.

Mike was a wrestler. When he channeled his temper in the right direction, it became a superpower. His only problem was his weight. He tended toward the stocky side until his height finally caught up with his weight several years later. In wrestling, there are different weight classes, and if you are as much as one pound over the limit at weigh-in, you get moved up into the next weight class, where someone could outweigh you by almost twelve pounds. That's an enormous advantage for your opponent when you're a teenage boy. Making weight became his obsession, and Mike was often running miles in plastic sweat suits, repeatedly spitting into a cup and, as a last resort, vomiting up any food until the necessary weigh-in number showed on the scale.

I watched him go from a chubby teenager to a slim young man within a few months, and it made a big impression on me. A growth spurt magnified his metamorphosis from boy to man, and he reached six feet before he stopped growing, but all I saw were his pounds melting away. It seemed like a magical power to me.

My brothers made puberty look easy, but when I reached the milestone, it wasn't so simple. I got made fun of for liking horses, felt awkward, and convinced myself I was unattractive. Several classmates teased me because I talked about horses all the time, calling me "horsey". If you are going to be teased for something, loving horses isn't all bad. But when they get up in your face day after day, they can make your life miserable.

A particular boy teased me in front of the class daily. He would stomp his feet, neigh like a horse, and snort in my face. After weeks of the teasing, I slapped him across the face. I glimpsed the teacher in my peripheral vision just as my hand landed on the boy's cheek, and he glanced away, as though he never witnessed the incident. The teacher knew that the boy deserved it. I'm sure he smiled to himself as the red imprint of my hand on the boy's face stopped my harasser from teasing me and warned others away from it for a good long while.

I went from a skinny kid to a shapely young woman, and I hated my new form. It felt like my body betrayed me. I wasn't ready to grow up; I wanted to stay in Never-Never Land, playing in my imaginary world, riding my horse, and finding fun every chance I got. But biology doesn't care what you want- it will do as it pleases despite your feelings.

My child-like body was lithe and reliable. It felt good; I liked it just the way it was. I detested the alien that seized my body, adding hair in personal places and curves that made my clothes too tight, and the bleeding once a month was an enormous inconvenience. What do you mean I can't go swimming? How am I supposed to ride my horse with this thick pad between my legs? I refused to stop enjoying the activities I loved. There had to be a way I could continue living my lifestyle.

There was- it was called a tampon. When I was young, we didn't have easy-glide plastic applicators. There was only one brand with a cardboard applicator, and the thing looked huge! The thought of inserting such a contraption up there was terrifying. My privates were an outlet for elimination only, right? Since we had one bathroom and my mom was not shy, I'd seen her insert tampons with ease. But I never imagined that I would ever need to do such things to *my* body.

My determination and stubbornness won out, and I locked myself in the bathroom with my mom's box of tampons. With the directions spread out on the counter, I read them repeatedly, hands shaking uncontrollably. With one foot on the toilet and my right hand on the tampon, I cried. Despite my mom's offer of support from outside the door, I refused to let her in. I was too embarrassed to let her help me. Driven by a strong will to do this myself- and even stronger desire to be free of those dreadful pads- I succeeded after a few tries.

A late bloomer, I was one of the last girls in my class to develop breasts. But when they showed up, they screamed, "Look at me!" My brothers used to call me "sweater girl" because when I wore a sweater, viewed from the side, I looked like I would tip over. It was like wearing a neon sign on your chest. They stuck out against my small body and drew attention everywhere I went. The girl that was once mistaken for a boy was now the object of conversation. At least that's what my brothers told me, that their friends were noticing.

"What? My sister? You think she's hot?"

I never thought I was hot, but strangely, I wanted to be. I was caught between being a woman and a child, with each one calling to me. Some days I would ride my horse from sun up to sun down, traveling 2.5 miles into town to ride with my horsey friends. We'd spent hours making up games which included racing through town, across manicured lawns, clip-clopping over brick covered streets and darting down gravel alleyways.

Then I'd ride back home, another 2.5 miles on a dead-tired Patches. I smelled like a horse, didn't bother with my hair, and felt happy. Other days, I wore too much make-up, tight sweaters and flirted with the boys. On those days, I didn't know who I was, what they expected of me, or how to behave, and I was miserable. I felt like I was out at sea with no compass. Still, I clung onto one world while reaching for the other.

I have since learned that being in this nowhere space, called transition, where one hasn't fully left one stage and yet has not integrated into the new, is the hardest part of life. Teetering between two worlds, trying to stand with one foot on either side of the line, is a precarious place to be.

Cultures that celebrate this passing from youth to adulthood through events like a quinceanera, a traditional coming of age celebration for Latina girls, understand the importance of creating a rite of passage to help everyone recognize such a major life change. In a quinceanera, when a Latin girl turns fifteen, her community holds an elaborate ceremony that highlights God, family and friends, and celebrates her transition with food, music and dancing. People treat these girls adorned in brightly colored dresses as if they were princesses. They celebrate her passage into womanhood, marking a clear distinction between one life and the next, encouraging her to leave the old and embrace the new, providing her with a mental bridge to cross over. In modern culture, at least the one I grew up in, families and communities are mostly void of such ceremonial events.

Some girls carry their weight well, but me, not so much. I have short arms and legs, narrow hips, and a small frame, so extra pounds show up quickly on me, especially in my face. Chubby cheeks, that's what I have. Apparently, I had chubby butt cheeks too. Because when I was in school, the humiliation of walking down the hall in front of high school boys as they laughed at my ass and made fun of me still burns.

While teenage boys grow taller, gain muscle, and consume more calories than ever, many teenage girls face a crushing blow. Their bodies prepare for childbearing by grabbing up calories like a Pac Man on steroids, storing it for the future.

I could no longer eat whatever I wanted and stay the same weight. Calories added up much faster. Gone were the days of eating one piece after another of warm toast, covered in butter and jam without thinking about it. Cellulite was the dreaded disease that resulted from such binges. Curdled cheese clinging to thighs, arms, and buttocks disgusted me. No wonder those boys made fun of me! I was fat, and that's all I could think of.

Food has taught me many things. The first lesson I learned was that we could use it as a control weapon. The second lesson I learned was how to use it as an emotional crutch, to "eat" my feelings instead of dealing with them. That's what I had watched my mom do. I began my own unhealthy relation-ships- first, with food, and later, with men.

Stuffing food down as fast as I could became a coping mecha-nism for me as a teenager. When I was upset or unhappy, I ate, just like my mom did. As a child, I ate when I was hungry and I stopped when I was full, and then I'd run off to some new adventure without putting much thought into what I consumed. But the strange new world that I entered as a teenager had different rules.

Every day, when I got dressed, or undressed, or every time my thighs rubbed together, or my jeans got tighter and had to be replaced with a larger size, I hated myself more. What the @$*! happened to me?

It's no wonder I sought to return to a childlike body. It's now clear to me I was trying to avoid growing up. Deep in my subconscious was the belief that staying in my childhood body would keep out the harsh realities of life. When things got too much to bear, I could saddle up my horse and ride away. My subconscious reasoned, if I lost enough weight, I could get my lithe body back and leave puberty.

So, I asked my brother to teach me how to throw up. If that magical power could transform him from a frog into a prince, perhaps it could help me look more like a princess instead of the awkward, chubby girl I had become. If I couldn't stop puberty, maybe I could beat it.

"How do you do that? Make yourself throw up?" I asked.

"It's easy, once you know the trick," he said.

"Will you teach me?" I asked.

He obliged, never realizing it would become a habit that would almost destroy my life. For him, it was a means to make weight. For me, what started as an experiment became an obsession. And it was NOT simply sticking your finger down your throat to provoke vomiting, as you might assume. I won't share the secret he taught me, because I never want to be responsible for such behavior. I don't blame my brother for my bulimia. It was my twisted thinking that brought on and kept me in my addiction.

The pain of life, the alien in my body, and an unhealthy relationship with food set me up for a lifelong struggle. Food was not my friend. That's what I had learned in my few short years on earth.

ELEVEN:

Practice makes perfect

In the beginning, vomiting wasn't the problem, but a solution. I needed an escape from the consequences of overeating. Perhaps, had I been part of a culture that celebrated my physical maturing instead of being teased and shamed over my weight, I may not have begun my path to self-destruction.

An unhealthy relationship with food, deep emotional pain, and a burning desire to reach perfection drove me into a world of eating disorder madness. I began by binge eating. In time, I adopted bulimia (purging by vomiting and/or laxative use). Eventually, I also embraced anorexia nervosa (restricting food intake which leads to low body weight, and is typically accompanied by an intense fear of gaining weight and a disturbed perception of body weight and image).

Bingeing for me was more than just overeating. I soon discovered that it becomes a demon, possessing its victim and taking them over.

Chocolate chip cookies were the trigger for me. Sugar, flour, butter, eggs, and chunks of chocolate are a few simple ingredients that are harmless until you combine them and they become cookie dough. Back then, sugar was a staple kept in ten-pound white and pink paper bags in the pantry. Every kitchen in rural Nebraska had them. For me, eating cookie dough was like eating legalized cocaine. Licking one sticky beater clean was never enough. That led to two beaters, licked clean. And then I ate one spoonful after another until half the batter was gone.

Then there were warm, gooey cookies dipped in cold milk. The satisfying crunch, as crumbs dribbled down my chin while I stood at the counter, stuffing my mouth with one cookie after another was addicting. Once the sugar rush began, it became a feeding frenzy. Like a blood-crazed piranha, there was no stopping me. At the height of a binge, my mind would remove itself from my body, as though I were watching someone else, until a bloated stomach brought me back to reality. And by then, it was too late.

If I thought being forced to eat an entire pizza had felt bad, this was worse. I did this to myself. My distended abdomen felt as though it would burst. That pain led to regret, which then turned to horror. Like the cookie dough, swirling around in a metal bowl, forced to submit to angry beaters, changing from ingredients into dough, my body took hold of my thoughts, and pain, regret, and horror spun around in my head until something had to give.

At first, making myself throw up was hard. But it got easier with practice. I learned cookie dough is easy to throw up, if you wash it down with milk. Cookies are harder to bring back up, but again, milk helps. Purging after a binge was like fast-forwarding past commercials. You get the good stuff and skip the things you don't like. It feels empowering and like any good drug, it makes you high.

The thought of hanging over a toilet, throwing up appalls most people. Memories of nausea, beads of sweat on their forehead, and painful retching are enough to drive them away from such a practice. Why would anyone do that to themselves?

I did it because vomiting by my method wasn't like that. I didn't feel nauseous, and there was no retching or pain- just relief, as all of those calories slid past my mouth into the abyss, like the binge had never even happened. One minute you are rolling around on your bed, holding your tummy, wishing you could take back the binge, and the next you are flying freely. And one good high lead to another.

I read that the stomach is the second brain, and so intimately connected are they that one affects the other. The brain sends signals or "talks" to the stomach and the stomach talks back.

Think of how your gut feels when you are anxious or upset, churning acid at a rapid pace, doing flip-flops and making you feel sick. Your brain communicates with all of your body, but the brain and the gut are like besties, sharing intimate details of not just a physical nature, but an emotional one as well.

They exchange more information between each other than do any other systems. In fact, only the brain has more nerve cells than the stomach. To put it simply, they feel one another's pain.

I wonder what they said to one another after a binge.

"What did you do to me?" asked the stomach. "All this food at once! Are you trying to kill me?"

"I didn't mean to hurt you. I blacked out and the next thing I know, all the cookies were gone," said the brain.

Stomach says, "They aren't gone. You dumped them on me!"

"I'm so sorry," said the brain, hanging her head.

"Ohhhh…do something. This hurts so bad!"

After such an early experience, the brain made sure we could empty contents of the stomach on command. The more you do something, the better you get at it, until it becomes a habit, or an addiction. And no one ever plans to get addicted. Not to drugs, alcohol, people, or harmful behaviors.

I didn't think about the consequences or the impact purging might have on my life until I couldn't stop it, which happened about the time I went to college. By then, purging was part of my routine, like brushing my teeth, or fixing my hair. It was part of who I was. But few people knew about it.

My family figured it out after I repeatedly left the table after eating and went immediately to the bathroom, but we rarely talked about it, or why I did it. Secrecy is part of the seduction. Making yourself throw up isn't something you do as a group activity or as a family outing. It's a solo thing. At first you lie about doing it because you feel ashamed. Then, you lie about doing it because people watch your every move, raise their eyebrows, or follow you to the bathroom. None of those behaviors stop you. In fact, I think they make things worse.

Being alone, lost in yourself and drowned by your emotion, is where you live when you have an eating disorder, and it is a very dangerous place to be. You lie to yourself, and there is no one to stop you from that deceit, and you believe everything you tell yourself.

"You are worthless."

"You're fat."

"You don't deserve good things."

However, to you, everyone else is the liar, and you don't trust them. That's where the illness takes over and you are no longer yourself or able to recognize truth from lies.

Initially, throwing up, binge eating or starving is a symptom, not the problem. Later, they become the problem, and many times, the focus for help. But when one starts, it's a symptom of much bigger issues. I couldn't have told you why I threw up or why I binged, not at age thirteen, or fifteen, or even eighteen. I can understand why now, but then, I didn't have a clue.

Eating was an escape from reality. It disconnected me from my body, my emotions, and myself, like an out-of-body experience. Once a binge was over, then shame set in. And then fear. Shame, from what I had done after promising myself I wouldn't do it again. And fear, of all the calories I just consumed, and overwhelmingly of getting fat.

My anxiety was insufferable until I purged. Throwing up was a relief, and to me, it felt good. It's crazy, right? Now that I understand the pattern. It is easy to see that I was stuffing my feelings inside, like the food I consumed, and then releasing them through vomiting, which gave me a short-term high. The problem is I never expressed my feelings or dealt with the pain I faced. All of that crap got pushed further and further down. By purging, I got a high, numbed my senses while getting my "fix," and became more and more detached from my own feelings.

There is escape in the acts of eating and the purging. By purging, instead of dealing with feelings, you stuff them all inside, and then release them, and you also escape the consequences of bingeing and an overly full stomach, which, given its pain and discomfort, would normally dissuade you from overdoing it again. Do you see why bingeing and purging creates such a dangerous cycle?

It's like being on a merry-go-round spinning out of control. The faster it rotates, the stronger the centrifugal forces are that hold you in place, until you can't get off the contraption.

TWELVE:

Hope

When my mom healed from her breakdown, she sought treatment for alcoholism. I don't recall how long she was away, but when she returned, the booze at home disappeared. She experienced enlightenment and frequently recited the serenity prayer.

"God, grant me the serenity to accept the things I cannot change, courage to change the things I can and wisdom to know the difference."

Still, she continued to choose unsavory men, usually drunks who abused her emotionally and physically. One rammed his car into hers in a drunken rage, totaling her new ride. She wasn't in the car, so that was a plus. He disappeared from our lives after that incident, which opened the door for others to come in. The one I remember the most was Mark. Tall, handsome, and thin as a rail, he could drink more beer than anyone I ever met. Cardboard cases stacked in our kitchen that held four six-packs, one case stacked upon the next, disappeared daily.

Mark was a great guy when he was sober. He taught me to drive a stick shift on the back country roads in his beat-up orange Toyota truck. No matter how many times I killed the engine, or tossed him out of his seat trying to change gears, he never lost his temper. But when he drank, he was mean. And he drank a lot. He was thin because he rarely ate, and he lived on booze. Our trailer walls bore the evidence of his tantrums, with holes where he put his fists through them. Not only did he destroy our home, but he also destroyed my faith in humanity when he went after my mom during his drunken episodes. I left the trailer every chance I could, calling a friend to come get me so I could escape the chaos.

Those years are now a blur, but then they went rapidly, yet gruesomely slow. My oldest brother, Jeff, graduated from high school and joined my Uncle Bill in Texas to work in cable TV, a move that destined him for financial success. During my junior year of high school, my mom moved to a new town, so I went with her. My brother Mike was a senior in high school then, and he stayed behind. I imagine my mom moved in order to survive financially, but leaving my brother to live on his own as a teenager seemed unwise to me. I didn't care- I was glad he wasn't coming with us- but I always felt it was a big mistake on her part.

At first, I was miserable leaving my hometown and friends, but when I saw the art department at my new school and met Mr.

Liska, the art teacher, my life changed. The town we moved to was about three times bigger than the small town of three thousand people we left. This school must have had a lot more money to spend, because the art department was huge! It was in a brand-new building attached to the high school, two rooms of space for creative expression. My old school had a small, drab room as an after-thought for art, and that teacher had very little inspiration to offer an up-and-coming artist.

My heart soared the first time Mr. Liska put my work on the board for everyone to admire. It was a pencil sketch of my family. He taught me what different number pencils could do, how to create shadows, depth, and how to shade. Who knew you needed so many pencils?

Of course, I had to have a bright blue art box, akin to a plastic tackle box, to keep my treasures in. Pencils ranging from #2 to #8, sticky erasers, paper shading tools, paints, brushes, and colored pencils filled it to the brim. It had my name on it, in permanent black marker. That box made me almost as happy as riding my horse (which I missed desperately). I had graduated from Patches the pony to Lucky the quarter horse over the years, but she was being kept at Mark's house, as he was still my mom's boyfriend, even though we were several hours away from him.

In this new place, I was no longer in my brothers' shadows. No one knew who they were, and they didn't care. Here, it was just me forging my own path. When I arrived in town, I was about ten pounds overweight, bingeing, vomiting, and depressed.

I then joined the theater group at my new high school and found my tribe. There were five of us that became inseparable: Paula, Damon, Doug, Mark, and me.

We were in both Drama and Speech class together. Paula was a born-again Christian after being a destructive, red-headed wild child. "Drugs or Jesus." After trying the first, she chose the second. We became fast friends, wore Jesus Saves buttons, and went to church together on Sundays. Born and raised in a Lutheran church, I had a strong faith and now, I had someone to share it with. We became the school evangelists, and we got made fun of a lot. But we had each other for support and just didn't care what anyone thought.

At lunch we would pile in her tiny Volkswagen truck and drive around blaring Bob Dylan's album, Saved. It put me on a much better track than where I'd been heading in my hometown. We didn't drink, smoke, or cuss.

Doug was tall, handsome, and had an incredible singing voice. It surprised none of us when he got the lead in the school musical, South Pacific. I tried out for the musical as well. We all did, except Damon. I could act, and they wanted to give me the lead female, Nellie, opposite of Doug, but I couldn't hold a tune in a basket, so I was cast as the sweet island girl, Liat. Mark got the part of Lieutenant Joseph Cable, who in the play, falls in love with Liat.

You would think Paula and I would fall for Doug, right? I always found tall men intimidating. Damon was Doug's best friend, a skinny geek with glasses and a friendly smile. I fell for the geek and Paula had a thing for Mark. Damon wasn't any good at acting or speaking, so he wasn't part of our weekend trips to school competitions, but that didn't stop us from dating and falling in love.

After they cast the four of us (Doug, Mark, Paula and I) in a one-act play, we formed even stronger friendships. We won several awards that year for our one-act play at state level competition, and I received a high honor for superior acting. I now had friends, a boyfriend, and a new purpose.

My grades went from C's and D's to A's and B's. I started researching art scholarships with Mr. Liska's help and encouragement. I felt happy for the first time since we had made the move. My bingeing was almost non-existent. However, I resorted to starving myself to lose weight after being made fun of by a group of popular boys. I'd go all day without eating, allowing myself one small meal after school. I soon dropped the extra pounds and became a sleek one hundred and ten pounds. For the first time in my teenage years, I felt attractive. Boys' heads turned, especially Damon's. They stopped making fun of me, and Damon pursued me with a passion.

Starving myself at first was hard. The gnawing hunger pains and light-headedness from my empty stomach were powerful, but not as powerful as the control I now held over and through my body. Like a shiny sword or a hefty gun, that control felt good in my hands. No one was making fun of me anymore.

The rewards of not eating outweighed the discomforts. And I felt like I belonged, had a bright future, and I liked myself. The better I felt about myself, the more my life improved.

The depressed, chubby girl turned into a swan. I received positive attention from teachers for my contributions in class, especially in art and English literature. Other kids would ask me to help them with their homework or art projects. Mr. Liska assisted me in researching art scholarships at various universities until I decided on the University of Northern Colorado as my first choice. My weight stayed steady, my bingeing and purging were minimal, and I smiled a lot. But I now had another weapon in my self-destructive arsenal- self-starvation. I had learned to control my hunger, something most people can't do, and that felt like a superpower that I could take out and use it if I ever needed to.

And then new bombs dropped.

First, my horse, Lucky, died. After we left the farm and couldn't keep our animals, my mom arranged for my horse to stay at Mark's house. Mark had acres of land which he had inherited from his family, so there was room to board my horse there. When Mark wasn't drunk, he farmed. Our move had taken us hours away from him, but my mom continued to see him on weekends.

The news of Lucky's death came to me while I was in the high school dressing room one evening preparing for our big night on stage. Why my mother decided to tell me about Lucky right before the big show still disturbs me. Why could she not wait until after the show?

The story was that Mark had tied Lucky up in a barn with a low roof, and for whatever reason, Lucky spooked, reared up, hit her head on a beam, and the blow killed her. I imagined that scene, playing it over in my mind, certain that Mark had been in a drunken rage and caused her death. That was more likely the truth. I went numb, but there was no time to process that news before going on stage that evening. I'm not sure I ever told any of my friends about it. It was too awful for me to believe, much less to talk about, but I carried a silent rage and deep sorrow in my heart from it for a long while.

My world exploded again when my mom lost her job and moved us back to Grand Island, Nebraska, for my senior year of high school. Everything I had worked for during the last year vanished, and my hope went with it. To start over my senior year at a new school sent me into the abyss. I was used to small town living. The school I attended at Grand Island had thousands of kids, drugs, and gangs. You didn't dare look at any of the boys at school because the girls would hurt you if they thought you were trying to move in on their territory. The girls had established cliques, and they weren't about to let any newcomers in.

I was alone again. I had no horse, no friends, and Damon had gone off to college, hundreds of miles away. The art classes at my new school sucked. There was no art department like I'd had, no Mr. Liska, no drama team filled with friendly faces, so I cut classes, until I wasn't even attending school any more. Instead, I'd go hang out with people much older than myself that I'd met while working as a server on the weekends. I worked in a popular bar/restaurant in the local mall, so most of the employees were over 21. You are who you hang with, and most of these people certainly weren't born-again Christians. They helped me get a fake I.D. so I could go bar hopping with them on the weekends. I never did drugs or smoked cigarettes, but booze? I drank my share when I was with them.

Damon and I were still seeing each other about once a month when I made a 2-hour trip to Lincoln. While attending college, he stayed with his grandparents and pursued a degree in Computer Science. He was my first love, my first lover, and I put all of my heart into our relationship since there was no one and nothing else for me to lean on.

College was where he thrived. The geek, once shunned in high school, became popular with the crowd that had humiliated him daily. He got rid of his pop bottle glasses with contacts, grew taller, and had me as a girlfriend. That gave him bragging rights, especially since we were having sex. As a Christian, it left me with guilt and shame, while he got pats on the back from his so-called friends.

Over time, phone calls from him became less frequent, and usually resulted in a fight, with me pleading and crying until I slipped into a lonely pit of darkness. I had gone on the birth control pill reluctantly. My doctor said sex was a natural thing, nothing to be ashamed of as he wrote out my script for the little white pill. The mini-pill, as it was called, had fewer hormones, less side effects, and apparently was less effective for young, fertile females. At that time, I never realized I'd had a miscarriage, and I don't recall the doctor ever telling me why he was prescribing all the pain medication, but the episode of bleeding and the pain, that I recall.

A final blow came when Damon and I broke up. I arrived at his grandparents' house to spend a weekend with him. After two hours in the car and weeks without seeing him, it surprised me that he was on the phone with one of his buddies when I arrived, and they were making plans for that evening. Not once was my name mentioned in that exchange. I sat in the hallway, my back against the wall, listening to the conversation, and I realized that he had no intention of spending time with me. A new resolve took over, and I quietly slipped out of the house, got in my car, and drove away.

I had several bottles of pain meds at my disposal, no clue about what had just happened in my body, and no reason to live. Years of being in chaos from my mom dealing with alcoholism and abusive boyfriends, making multiple moves, and having damaged self-esteem from my malicious brothers landed me at the bottom of a well.

Escape from the pain. That was all I could think of. And there was one way out, according to my brain, so I took a handful of pills and went to sleep. I never wanted to wake up again. But I did. My body is highly sensitive, just like my spirit, and it purged the poison before I passed into oblivion. Damn body- I hate you. Why won't you let me leave?

The main thing I recall about being in the hospital following my suicide attempt was how adamant I was that my dad could not come see me. I recall that, and sleeping for days. The medical staff kept me sedated, and I recall little. My mom came to see me, but I refused to see my dad.

It took me years to figure out why I didn't want to see my dad. I was too ashamed, and I couldn't face him. No matter what happened or what I did, I always knew that my mom would still love me, but this was not so with my dad. He did not state this to me, but his actions taught me that his love for me was conditional.

Then was the first time that I worked with a counselor, and the man I worked with wasn't a very good one. I don't recall our conversations, but I can tell you he never got through my steeled heart to the truth, - not even close. I wish someone would have asked me the one thing that got swept under the rug, "Why did you try to kill yourself?" Ask me for the truth, right out. Maybe they did, but I don't remember it. By not asking me the hard question, it allowed me to conceal the truth from myself.

Like a totem pole, I had become one character stacked on top of the next, a person of multiple faces, but lacking understanding of what each figure I conveyed represented. I binged, purged, starved, and did not know who I was, where I was going, or what made me happy.

But one thing was for certain: I was angry and I would not talk about it. Not to my mom, not to my counselor, not to my so-called friends. I was tightly shut up, keeping my heart hard and my mouth closed.

THIRTEEN:

Flailing

My counselor suggested I change schools. There was a smaller high school I could attend in town, and we decided I would finish my senior year there. I might have flourished in that new environment, but it was too late in the year for me to accomplish much. I'd stopped caring about my future or my art scholarship, had few new friends, and I continued to skip school.

Things came to a head one day between my mom and me. She didn't know I was harboring such anger. I don't remember what I called her at the dinner table, but it was bad enough to cause her to slam my head into the wall three times before I left the house. She did not tolerate a lack of respect, and such language was never to be used.

My dad said I could come live with them for a while, so I packed my stuff and left since they lived only a half-hour away. That didn't last long, as being in such a foreign environment only made me feel worse. It served as a good cooling-off period for my mom and I, though, and I returned home after several weeks. I quit attending school until my counselor suggested I finish midterm. My credits sufficed, allowing me to graduate early.

Before I could graduate, there were finals I needed to complete. A passing grade would do, so I hurried through them as fast as possible. The teacher administering the tests surprised me. Not only was she kind, but she said something I still cherish.

"Cynthia, I have never had a student complete the tests so quickly and get such high scores. What are you doing? You should go to college."

"What?" I asked.

"You are smart and should apply for college."

"You really think so?" I asked.

"Yes, I do. Think about it."

That was the first time anyone ever told me I was smart, besides my mom, but she didn't count. Moms always said that stuff. I had struggled with math, so they tried to put me in summer school one year, but I never made that class because it was the summer my mom and D.R. got divorced and we moved. They might have caught my learning disability then; instead, I thought I was stupid. Now I realize I have dyslexia with numbers, often turning them around, mixing them up. No wonder I got D's in math, struggled to understand the concepts, and fell behind in my math classes.

Reading and writing I could do, often flourishing when I applied myself. But numbers confused my brain. My brother Mike, for all his faults, spent hours teaching me to tell time and count change. He was the only one with the patience. We'd sit on the floor, a jar filled with change, or a clock, while he repeated the lessons many times before I grasped the concepts.

I shrugged off the idea of college, but her words had a tremendous impact on me. It took only one person to plant a positive thought in my mind and build my confidence.

The summer after I graduated from high school, I moved out. Years of living with my mom's chain smoking, repressed anger inside, and an independent spirit pushed me out of the nest. My mom never let on that it was hard on her, but not long after I moved out, she took off for Wyoming, a place where she had dreamed of living. I'm sure an empty nest helped push her toward a new life of her own.

Fall was coming up fast, and with it, everyone I knew was preparing to go off to college while I worked two server jobs to support myself. I panicked at the thought of being left behind, so at the last minute, I applied to the University of Nebraska, Lincoln, where most of my old friends were going. Luckily, I was admitted and I enrolled.

It was not a move I put a lot of thought into, and in my mental condition, I had no business attending college, taking a full load of classes. I don't think I had a mental illness then. I think I had a mental wound, and I didn't know how to heal it. Pain cut my soul so deep that it bled out into every area of my life. But the stress of college, along with lack of financial and emotional support, pushed me to a new level of self-destruction.

A college campus is rife with triggers for someone with an eating disorder. It's hard enough for an emotionally healthy individual to stay balanced that first year in the academic world, but for me, it was impossible. My perfectionism applied not only to myself but also to my grades. I had a new goal: to make the Dean's list.

At first, everything about college life was exciting, sending a rush of good feeling hormones throughout my body. When the drudge emerged and the pressure mounted, not only from my class load but also from my lack of financial help, my disorder took over. With a meal card, a smorgasbord of food choices in the cafeteria, and no restrictions, I grew into a human bingeing and purging machine. Anything left in my stomach after vomiting got dealt with harshly by laxatives. I knew where every bathroom on campus was.

Bulimics are usually normal to slightly above-average in weight. Vomiting is not a very effective weight-loss tool; at least it wasn't for me. It did, however, serve the purpose of controlling the after effects of binge eating. That, and laxative abuse, kept me at an average weight and from gaining the "Freshman Ten." That's what people called the ten pounds a college freshman usually gains their first year, and it's no wonder.

Eating pizza at midnight, watching afternoon soap operas between classes lounging on beanbag chairs, and having access
to an all-you-can-eat buffet style cafeteria with the swipe of
a card can cause weight gain and unhealthy eating habits. If
you didn't have an eating disorder before you came to college,
the chance you'd develop one before you graduated was pretty
high. When young adults are removed from their family structure and given free rein in the campus cafeteria, it can lead to
disastrous results. As a freshman in the dormitory, I purchased
a meal card for the semester, which allowed for three meals a
day in any of the campus cafeterias. It was like an all you can
eat buffet. Mounds of food with a large variety of choices including a desert bar and ice cream bar were spread before us.
No shopping, no food prep, and no thought had to go into your
meals. You just show up and eat, like a pack of lions in the zoo.

All of it was addicting. The endless mounds of food, late-night
pizza parties and the vomiting afterwards. Stress caused by
living in proximity with people you don't know, class loads with
endless homework, peer pressure to drink, smoke and get high,
not to mention the sex scene. When I was in college, co-ed
dorms had just started. Boys lived on one end, girls on the
other, and parties in the middle.

Young adults with underdeveloped frontal lobes living away
from their families for the first time, with little or no supervision, were set up for disaster. Even if you came from a family
with loose morals and few rules, at least you had some sense
of community at home. Here, on campus, anything went. If

you were raised in a strict household, the consequences could be even broader.

Suddenly, no one was watching what you did, and your peers didn't care. Party hard. That was the only rule. The teachers didn't care if you showed up for class, as long as someone paid the tuition. We weren't in Kansas (or Nebraska) anymore, Dorothy. No hall passes were required to get out of classes, no forged signatures with lame excuses needed. This was the college world I entered over forty years ago. I can't imagine what it's like now. No wonder suicide, drug addiction, and alcohol poisoning take so many young lives.

We think freedom is the answer- freedom from rules, boundaries, parents, siblings, teachers. Free sex, the more the merrier. No one gets hurt, as long as we all have fun, and it feels good, right? I believe that this is our mental health crisis in America and it's only going to get worse. History shows that the more rope we have, the faster most of us hang ourselves.

Left to themselves with underdeveloped brains, over-developed sex drives, and little or no adult supervision, young adults on college campuses face huge temptations. Many college kids make games out of drinking, as though the drunker you are, the cooler you get. In reality, the drunker you are, the dumber you look. But if everyone else is drunk too, it's funny- until it's not, when someone gets raped, overdoses, or dies.

I didn't drink, smoke, or have sex in college. I studied all hours of the day and night, binged, purged and self-destructed without any of those other indulgences to blame. My poison was different, but no less addicting.

Without many rules or healthy boundaries in college, I made up my own. It is there where I decided I liked rules, and the more rules I made for myself, the more in control I felt. Life in my family had taught me that others get to control you. Here, no one controlled me, so I had to do it myself. I started counting calories until I knew the amount for every food item I ate, and I developed a list of "bad" foods. The list grew daily, and I bounced between not eating at all, avoiding my ever-growing list of forbidden foods, to binge eating and purging into the night, until nothing stayed in my stomach- not even a cup of coffee.

Mental illness happens after years spent in an eating disorder. When your mind becomes twisted and you've spent so many years telling yourself lies, your thoughts are no longer realistic, but you believe they are the truth. Lies become your reality. My world consisted of studying daily into the night, drinking coffee to stay awake, purging, and diving behind buildings to throw up if a bathroom wasn't close by. I believe I had reached mental illness at that time.

When you are in the depth of despair, your mind twisted like a pretzel, you have little sense of normalcy. I'd spent so many years tied in knots, I didn't know what normal was. Is there such a thing? Somewhere, deep down, I wanted help.

FOURTEEN:

Self-Discovery

As a student, one perk was access to free counseling. I made an appointment, unsure if anyone would understand what I was going through. The counselor I met was soft-spoken, direct, and I liked her. Though I don't remember her name, I remember some of our conversations.

During one session, she stopped me while I was telling about my life growing up.

"Cynthia, you're smiling," she said.

"What?" I asked.

"You are describing an incredibly painful event, but you are smiling. Did you know that?"

I didn't know that. And it was weird.

"Why do you think you do that?" she asked.

She asked me the hard questions, and I respected her for it.

"Well, fuck," is what I wanted to say.

How long had I been doing that, smiling when I should have been crying? She didn't need to ask me that question. I got to that one on my own.

We talked about my past during our twice weekly sessions. I relived my childhood, describing what happened, and how I felt.

"Do you realize that your life has been chaos since your mom and dad got divorced?" she asked.

"What?" I asked. That thought had never crossed my mind.

"You have gone from one chaotic situation to another. Every time life evened out, the rug got pulled out from under you."

I'd lived in it for so long, chaos was normal to me.

Double fuck.

"I want you to keep a journal," she said. "I think it will help."

Entries of a few words at first eventually turned into full pages, and soon, the journal filled up. Each week, I'd read her some of my entries, opening new discussions.

One day, the topic of the death of my horse, Lucky, came up. I controlled a smile as I told her the story.

"That was a defining moment for you, wasn't it?" she asked.

She not only saw my pain, but she felt it.

Nodding my head, with tears dripping off my nose, I sobbed. Releasing the pain in her office that day was a milestone. It still brings tears to my eyes today as I write these words. After all these years, that memory still hurts. I think the body remembers trauma long after it is over- not just the mind, but the body. You can choose to let things go, convince yourself it's in the past, talk positively to yourself, but your DNA remembers. Just like in me reliving that counseling memory now, the pain remains.

The difference between being happy and miserable, though, is whether we choose to dwell on the pain. We get to decide how long we savor feelings, good or bad, and that is where the magic lies. Which is what my counselor tried to teach me. Recognize, release, refuse.

Recognize what happened and how it made you feel.

Release the pain. Talk, scream, cry- but let it out.

Refuse to allow it to dwell in your mind. And when it comes back up, you can say to yourself, "I already dealt with that. I'm not allowing the past to ruin my present."

But I would not learn to effectively use the three R's until much later in life. And it took years of practice for me to undo what had been done. Life had become so painful for me, I lived pretending everything was fine. That is my truth. I lived hiding from my feelings because they were too painful to face, and that's why I put a smile on my face. My body had learned to lie not only to myself, but to others.

An eating disorder, no matter how you label it, is all about lies. And secrecy. You lie to yourself about yourself until you believe those lies, and then you lie to others. And you live bingeing, purging, or starving in silence.

Counselors, psychiatrists, and therapists love to label things, creating names, terms and tags for conditions, such as anorexia nervosa, bulimia, bulimarexia…blah, blah, blah. The list of names has grown over the years, and now it's more confusing than ever.

When I was growing up, anorexia nervosa was the thing people were talking about, and it became big news when it claimed the unforgettable life and voice of Karen Carpenter. Bulimia and bulimarexia were just emerging as eating disorders. That doesn't mean they hadn't existed before- but rather, they were being recognized and labeled. No matter what label somebody gave me or I attached to myself, I was messed up, and my situation only got worse.

Eating disorders gained prominence at a time in history when being mentally ill was the same as being crazy. At least, that's what I thought. I subscribed to many labels, but being crazy wasn't one of them. Who gets to decide if someone is crazy? And are all such diagnoses correct because a professional says so? Are you mentally ill and then you develop an eating disorder? Or do you have an eating disorder and become mentally ill? Does that make you crazy, too? I wish I would have asked these questions. And I wish they would have discussed such things openly with me.

Can you be mentally ill and not be crazy? I think so. This is the space I occupied for a long time. I would like to have seen the notes and diagnosis counselors gave me, but no one ever said such things to my face. They whispered to my parents, or perhaps to each other, but never to me. Charts hung at the bottom of my bed in the hospital scribbled with notes, but I never dared to read them because that's the way it was back then.

I'm sure those pages were covered in words describing my disease of the mind that now manifested itself in my body. Then, the person living the crisis seemed to be the only person with whom such things weren't discussed. Do you see the irony? That was the kind of treatment I received. Advancements in medicine for the mind and the body have developed, and there is now treatment for the entire family, as well as in-patient, out-patient, and group therapy available in facilities for various eating disorders.

We have come a long way in disorder diagnoses and treatment, but the person in the disorder is the only one who really knows what goes on in their mind. And by the time they recognize it and can or will discuss it with others, their life may be in jeopardy. Based on my experience, the chances of healing are greater when addressing such behaviors early.

Honest discussions with me by doctors, psychiatrists and counselors were what I wished had happened, not with my family, who were part of the problem. My college counselor was one of the best I ever had. She was years ahead of most professionals, but even she skirted around issues.

Most of my journal entries were not profound. Because my mind dwelled on food, I wrote often about what foods I could or would eat, and what foods I wouldn't. I kept my exhaustive lists of good or bad foods, and the bad list grew daily (good foods were foods I would eat, and bad foods were foods I refused to eat). I logged how many calories I'd consumed, how often I binged and threw up, and I chronicled page after page about my obsession with my weight and feeling fat.

That semester in college, I teetered between binge eating, purging and starving, depending on what the scale said. I was as determined to reach one-hundred pounds as I was to make the Dean's list. When I got close to that one-hundred-pound mark, I set a new goal of ninety-five.

My counselor did a smart thing. She said I wasn't "allowed" to drop below a hundred pounds. Who did she think she was? She wasn't my parent, my doctor or my friend. But I respected her. And I did as she said, no matter how badly I wanted to lose more weight. She was wise and gave me some leeway, but didn't allow me to hang myself. I could be a little underweight, but there was a line she said I couldn't cross. And I never did. Not as long as she was my counselor, anyway.

We continued to meet the rest of the semester. I don't recall talking with her about much except my childhood drama and my obsession with food.

It's too bad I was so messed up that I missed the obvious in college- a lighted path that might have led me to a successful career. As a freshman, I took the required courses, but also one elective, and it was that elective course I enjoyed the most. It was also the class that came the easiest to me. Creative writing.

All those books I'd devoured as a child paid off in that writing class. I was a natural. We were required to share our assignments in class, taking turns reading our work out loud. Most of the class struggled with creative ideas for our weekly assignments. Not me. I had an endless stream of stories to tell. All I needed was a prompt from the teacher. After several weeks of reading my work to the class, one classmate spoke up.

"I always feel like I should applaud when you finish reading," he said in front of the class.

Too embarrassed to say anything back, I just sat there. The teacher acknowledged his comment and added his own.

"Yes," he said. "You are good enough to get published."

I've harkened back to their words many times. Part of me always knew I wanted to be a writer, but another side of me was so out of touch it did not know what I wanted. My eating disorder overshadowed the bright future I might have had as an author.

When it took over, it ruled my life, my future, and my decisions.

That's what any form of addiction does. It takes one piece of you at a time until there is nothing left of you but the disease. Addictions are greedy and they don't care what you want, where you want to go, or who they hurt.

I dropped out of college after one semester, unable to withstand the financial and emotional pressure. I'd made the Dean's list, just like I had strived for, but it came at a high cost.

Now I was a quitter. More lost than when I had started college, I moved out of the dorm and in with some friends, landing a dead-end job as a hostess in a local restaurant. My friends were all attending college, living together in a big house, so one more roommate in the basement was less rent for them to pay. No one cared if I was in school or not, just that I paid my share of the rent on time.

What they eventually did care about was finding the person who was raiding the food, and it took a while for me to be discovered. I started slowly, taking what seemed to be my fair share of food so that no one would notice. But they had busy lives, futures to build and studying to do. Me, I had a shitty job and an eating disorder.

One boy living in the house was from a big family, and he had a mama that loved to cook. She made all kinds of delicious treats- cookies, brownies, home-made granola, trail mix and fresh bread- for him, and there was enough for him to share, so his goodies lined the counters and filled the refrigerator. My roommates left each morning, departing in different directions, returning later at various times of the day. Left alone in a big house with nothing but my addiction and a kitchen of tempting treats, my fair share soon turned into a feeding frenzy.

I had every intention of having a handful, a spoonful, or a bite of one of those treats, but once I started plundering, I couldn't stop until the bag or plastic container was empty and the toilet was full. Do I keep the empties or throw them away? I'd stand at the counter, holding an empty plastic bag that minutes ago was full, and shame washed over me. I knew when my roommates came home, one-by-one, the first thing they would do was head to the kitchen. What I wanted to do was run away- from this house, my life, my eating disorder, and myself. But I had nowhere to go.

So, I lied.

"Who ate all the granola?" said one of my roommates as I was passing by. "This bag was full this morning."

"I don't know," I said as I shrugged my shoulders. "I was gone all day."

Each time I got away with it, I felt a little worse about myself. Now, guilt piled up on top of shame. You would think those feelings would stop me, but they didn't. The worse I felt about myself, the more I binged, raiding the personal stash of others. If it was in the kitchen, it wasn't safe around me.

I lived in the basement, so I'd slink into the darkness below and hide until each storm passed, not coming out except to leave for work. Accusations, heated arguments, and slammed doors occurred almost daily. People were pissed and suspected each other. I became depressed and slept a lot. For someone who had never been a good sleeper, that was a sign. All I wanted to do was crawl under the covers. It was hard for me to make it to work, let alone to do anything else. I'd wake up at night, after sleeping most of the day, and sneak into the kitchen. And that's how I got caught.

One of my roommates walked in on me, around two one morning, as I was dipping my wet fingers into a baggie of his mom's homemade granola, shoveling bite after bite in my mouth. Crumbs scattered all over the floor, the counter, and stuck to the sides of my mouth.

Disgust written all over his face, he was too mad to speak, too religious to cuss. I knew, without him saying a word, that I had to move out. I'd crossed an unspoken boundary and there was no going back.

When I left college, I had left my counselor and any shred of sanity I had. At our last meeting, she asked if she could keep my journal. I thought that was a strange request. But there was no good reason I shouldn't let her. It meant nothing to me. Just page after page of my obsession with food and my weight. Why would anyone want to read this crap? Now I see it must have been fascinating. I often wish I'd kept it, to read my thought processes, which is surely why she wanted to keep it, to study the thought patterns of someone with an eating disorder.

I never returned to college. While other kids my age were creating their future, I was throwing mine up.

There was one relationship I wish I'd been able to explore. I had met a soft-spoken, dark-haired and kind guy in one of my classes who liked to read as much as I did and we often spent hours discussing a book, life, and far-away places. While other boys tried luring me into their beds, he became my friend. I never told him my dark secret, but I wanted to. We never even kissed. I knew he was too good for me, that I didn't deserve this young man. So, I left him when I left college.

I'd lay awake at night and think about him, wondering what our relationship might have become if I didn't have an eating disorder. He was one of the few quality men I had met throughout my life, and I flushed him away.

FIFTEEN:

Survival Young Adult years

Survival mode is what I knew, and I spent the next seven years surviving instead of thriving.

On the one hand, I was mature well beyond my years. Because I grew up living in an alcoholic household and was often the parent instead of the child, I became codependent, playing the roles of caretaker and decision maker. I felt responsible for everything that happened and tried to fix it, apologizing all the time. I worked harder than most adults, believing that the world rested on my shoulders, doing what I felt I had to do. And yet, at times, I resorted to child-like behavior, seeking solace from a worn-out stuffed animal, and looking for someone to rescue me. I needed help, but I did not know what to do.

The problem is, when life happens, there is no ticket off of the ride. As an adult, the world comes at you with full force, and it will run you over. When you have to pay the rent, buy food, and care for others, fixing yourself is the last thing on the list. This is survival mode: getting by from one moment or one day to the next, doing whatever it takes.

I lived in survival mode most of my life, struggling to make ends meet, in one poor relationship after another, trying to fix everyone else when I was the one needing to be fixed. I worked at jobs I never liked but had to keep in order to live.

When I moved out of the big house with all of the roommates, I left Nebraska too. My mom was working as a secretary on a secluded ranch in Wyoming, living a life she'd dreamed about. Surrounded by mountains, horses and cowboys, she wisely chose for a partner a pilot she had met along the way. But before they married and he swept her away, she invited me to come visit.

I drove the thirteen hours from Nebraska to my mom's place straight through, arriving in the small mountain town exhausted but thrilled at my new surroundings. That cowboy town was just what this girl needed, and my two-week vacation turned into thirty years.

One day I was in a busy city, surrounded by tall buildings, people and chaos. The next, I was surrounded by mountains, few people and wide-open spaces. I found the best parts of myself again, riding along a mountain trail on horseback, alone for hours. Breathing in the fresh air, listening to nothing but the clip-clop of my horses' hooves on the rocky trails. It was a piece of heaven and I knew I wanted to stay.

My chance came when the ranch cook stopped showing up and lay passed out in his room. They needed me. They just didn't know it yet.

I convinced the ranch manager to give me a chance. Because I was only nineteen years old, he didn't think I had what it took to put three square meals a day on the table for up to twenty people. I had long ago learned to cook, though, often putting meals on the table for my family and I was confident I could handle the job.

"You have nothing to lose," I said. "Your cook is a drunk. Let me show you what I can do."

He looked at me with skeptical eyes and pursed lips. But he was thinking about it.

"Give me a week and let me prove it," I said, hands on my hips. "It'll take at least that long for you to find a replacement. If I can't do it, you can hire someone else and I'll go home."

By the end of the week, the drunken cook was gone, and I had taken over his room off of the kitchen. I worked six days a week, and for pay I got a small stipend plus room and board, with access to all the ranch horses, except for one- Steel. He was a black Morgan cross with wild eyes, and the ranch manager was the only one allowed to ride him.

"Give me one chance and let me prove I can ride him," I asked repeatedly.

And I did.

Steel and I became inseparable, and when the ranch manager handed the reins over to me, I was the only one allowed to ride the wild beast. That horse saved my life several times on the trail. He was sure-footed, had the energy of three horses, and a sixth sense for trouble. He warned me when a grizzly bear was following us, pulled a string of mules up a steep, mud-covered trail with me at the back, holding onto a mule's tail, and got us across solid ice on the side of a mountain that cost several horses their lives.

The ranch for me, was a paradise. Located at the end of an hour's drive outside of Cody, Wyoming, and inside the east gate of Yellowstone National Park it was untamed, incredibly beautiful and just what this cowgirl needed. While other kids my age were attending college, creating their future, I was riding horses, cooking meals for the ranch hands, and sleeping on the ground in a white canvas tent on pack trips.

"Wherever you go, there you are."

I don't know who said it, but I understand those words after living it for years. Changing physical circumstances did not change me or my behavior.

Working in a kitchen full-time was like putting a fox in charge of the henhouse. All that food was at my disposal, and I didn't have to pay the grocery bill. For a while, I kept myself in check, careful not to blow my cover. I was good at hiding from the truth, and I stayed on a budget month after month, despite my periodic binges.

"Where did all the cookies go?" asked one of the ranch hands. "There were dozens here just an hour ago."

"Must have been one hungry, hombre," I replied, smiling back.

The only person on the ranch who knew my secret was a new ranch secretary. As the only other girl working full-time on the ranch, we became quick friends, so she never gave me away.

She liked to ride and was an accomplished horsewoman. She eventually picked a sturdy white horse from the ranch herd, while I rode Steel, the black one. The contrast of our black and white horses was comical to everyone on the ranch. I'd saddle up both horses, and wait outside the ranch office until she got off work.

After my mom left, I needed a friend, and that she liked horses was enough to push me into action. I knew she couldn't say no if her horse was ready and all she had to do was climb on, so I made myself a nuisance with a smile she couldn't resist.

When she closed the office door, I'd hand over the reins to her white steed. She, too, was hiding from a painful past, and it took a lot of convincing on my part to get her to have some fun.

Streaks of black and white tore through the ranch and, on more than one occasion, we got in trouble. The ranch was owned by a rich family and featured trimmed lawns, tidy cabins, and the big house where the owners stayed was kept immaculate. A millionaire bachelor was hardly ever there, but when he was, he expected peace and quiet. There was no humor for him in two young ladies whooping and hollering, tearing through his yard. He liked to photograph wildlife and spent hours setting up his tripod for the perfect shot, and our shenanigans often ruined his efforts. He was young, available- and a spoiled brat. For our exploits, he'd scream at our backs and threaten to fire us. While he was present, we'd follow the rules, but as soon as he drove off the ranch, our fun resumed.

The ranch manager mentioned frequently that one of us should make a play for him. I had no use for bad-tempered money, and never gave the idea a second thought. Besides, he was geeky and wore the same boring beige pants and white shirt every day of the week. I once peeked in his closet and saw rows of identical clothes lined up in it. We all had a good laugh when I told the others about that.

Because my friend never liked to ride in the mountains, we spent our time in the saddle close to the ranch. I, however, was wild and adventurous and could never get enough of the majestic peaks. So, when the manager gave me an opportunity to be camp cook during hunting season, I jumped on it. The cook they had used for years was pregnant and unavailable.

While I was in the hills, they hired a temporary cook to feed the ranch hands. That was the closest I got to being found out.

After being up in the mountains for a week at a time, I'd return for a couple days and raid the cookie jar or pantry for other goodies she baked. It soon became obvious who was devouring the treats. She didn't take so kindly to her snacks disappearing, and I never understood why she was cross with me until my friend told me.

"Cynthia, she doesn't know you throw up. All she knows is you eat everything in sight and she can't keep up with you. Besides, she knows you are coming back to take her job away when hunting season is over. So don't expect her to like you."

That explanation didn't stop me, but for a spell, it slowed me down. I felt bad about eating all her hard work, but, once again, it didn't stop the bingeing and purging.

It was during my time on the ranch that I discovered I had a control issue. I kept a spotless kitchen and took great pride in keeping things clean. We all worked six days a week with just one day off. When my time away from the kitchen came, I'd saddle up Steel and disappear with a sack lunch into the mountains. We could cover a lot of miles together, as he was high-spirited and moved fast. There were so many uncharted trails to discover, and I wanted to ride all of them. We would return before dark, dragging our butts back to the barn, bone-tired but happy. Both of us had a spirit for adventure and I loved that horse. I still keep his picture on my bulletin board to remind me of his indomitable spirit.

While I was away from my duties, the ranch hands had to fend for themselves. One day a week, my kitchen was a free-for-all. I loved my day off, but I hated to come back to the mess. There were grease splatters on the stove; counter tops were not wiped clean; mud was tracked across my kitchen floor. Their untidiness sent me into a rage. They did the best they could with the short time they had on lunch or breaks, but it was never good enough. One day I got so mad, I stood on top of a chair and yelled at them. I thought I was well within my rights, but once again, my friend set me straight.

"Cynthia, don't you think you overreacted?"

"No, I don't," I replied

"They don't have time to clean the way you do. When you're out, they have to fix their own meals and clean up. Give them a break. They try, but they aren't perfect."

There it was again. Perfectionism. Now I'd pushed it on others, expecting them to hold to my strict standards. When my kitchen was clean, I felt in control. If one thing was out of place, I lost control.

Paradise lasted for two years until I met a man that worked temporarily on the ranch. I left the ranch to move in with him. We got married, and I had my first child. I threw myself into parenting with the same gusto as I did everything. I was all in.

When my first child arrived, it changed me. She gave me a reason to become healthy. During my pregnancy, I stopped bingeing and purging, and I focused on my growing child. I ate healthy, took good care of myself, and only threw up from morning sickness, which lasted off and on the entire nine months. My doctor suggested our unhappy marriage might be the reason for my affliction.

My husband was fourteen years my elder, but not much more mature than I. He was in a mid-life crisis, an abuser, and he was my first introduction to a narcissist. I didn't even know what a narcissist was when we met, but I memorized their behavior patterns by the time I left him for good. It took many tries on my part to get away completely, as he would manipulate, beg, or use control tactics to get me to come back.

The day he got an inch from my face and screamed "Shut the fuck up!" I could see it in his eyes. If I stayed with him, he would abuse me physically, like he did his ex-wife. He blamed her for everything that went wrong in his life. She was a bitch, and it was all her fault. My failure was believing him, until the tables turned on me, and by that time, my daughter had been born.

I mentally left the relationship the moment he screamed in my face, and I knew he was threatening me, and it was a taste of things to come. I would do whatever I had to for my daughter, to keep her safe, so I lied my way out of the relationship.

He hadn't held a steady job in over a year. He begged and borrowed his way from one bad situation to another and drug me along with him. When I was working, I had some power, but now I had a child to care for and depending on him, and he hadn't worked for months.

It's the most helpless feeling I've ever experienced. I had no car, no money, and he often left me alone for weeks while he ran off seeking his fortune, promising to drag us along on yet another dead-end road.

I begged him to drop me off at my mom's house in Casper, Wyoming, on our way to the next destination and promised to join him once he had a job and a place to live. Big lie. I had no intention of ever living with him again. My mom found me a counselor, helped me get to the legal aid office where I filed for divorce, and let me stay with her and her new husband for a few months while I got on my feet. With no college degree, few employable skills, and a child to take care of, I landed a low-paying job as a dental assistant and was in survival mode again.

I was young, ambitious, and optimistic, and I might have found a decent career if I'd had some help, but he ran off, and the child support never came. The meager amount we had agreed upon in the divorce went with him to Australia. He paid me once, but the check bounced, leaving me overdrawn with a sick child, begging the bank to forgive the fee. That $20 overdraft charge would pay for my daughter's medicine, so I begged them to forgive it.

He fled, leaving his obligations not just to us, but to a previous family, behind, evading child-support for twenty-six years, and leaving me to care for our daughter. His leaving was a blessing. I was finally free of his manipulation and control, but I never planned on raising a child alone. I was ill-prepared for the financial responsibilities of parenting and I struggled to provide for our basics.

He did much damage to me emotionally while we were together, and my bingeing and purging returned after my daughter came along. He knew about my vomiting and likened it to cheating on him. Every day, he'd ask if I threw up. I had to admit my failure to him when he came in the door and he'd brandish me verbally. If I loved him, I'd stop. He was manipulative, mean, and he shamed me often.

He was also sexually abusive, which I won't talk about to this day. I've told no one about what took place in our bedroom and I probably never will. I put it all behind me when he left, swearing that I'd never discuss the awful things he made me do. It happened so many years ago, so I don't feel the need for therapy, but I wish I would have opened up to a therapist and worked through that abuse. It would have saved me years of depression and more self-destruction.

The one good thing he gave me, besides my daughter, was a gym membership. A couple of years before I got pregnant, he'd given me a membership to the local gym, commenting that I had the right physique for a bodybuilder. Women's bodybuilding was in its infant stages, but it was big enough to attract me to the lifestyle. For the first time since my eating disorder began, I had a healthy goal- to look like one of the top stars. Forty years ago, female body-builders were shapely and feminine. My idol was Rachel McLish, a very sexy yet muscular woman, and I wanted to look like her. The extreme muscularity popular today was not the standard then, nor was the use of steroids.

I went from starving or purging to being obsessed about what I ate so I could fuel my workouts. You can't build muscle if you don't eat. I read about bodybuilding, studied what to eat, and changed my diet radically. Lifting weights was a positive outlet for my perfectionism. I kept pictures of my idols visible to remind me of the body I wanted. Instead of eating less, I ate more, but mainly lean protein sources like chicken and tuna. For the first time in years, food remained in my stomach. And my body reacted wildly. My dormant system came alive as I raced for the bathroom, but this time it wasn't laxatives that sent me running.

On some level, it was exchanging one obsession for another. But it was a start down the road of recovery. Lifting weights gave me a purpose, something else to think about. It also gave me a positive way to change the way I looked. I finally discovered a secret that I'd kept from myself:

I didn't like my body.

Most obsessive-compulsive disorders begin with fear and anxiety, much like my purging. Shame and guilt follow. Compulsive behaviors usually increase in times of increased stress or change, and often shift from one perceived threat to another, as though the brain needs something to worry about. Luckily, in my new routine, my focus went from starving to eating the right foods so I could build muscle. The desire to control my world with self-destruction shifted to a positive outlet.

Muscle burns more calories than fat, speeding up the body's metabolism. The more muscle you have, the more calories you need. Bodybuilding took self-discipline, focus, and hard work, which kept my mind busy, and the muscle I built created a high metabolism that increased as I aged. Instead of starving myself to be thin, my body burned calories faster, leaving me lean without deprivation.

It is hard to admit not being comfortable in your own skin- at least it was for me. The feelings I had about my body became how I felt about myself. Working out gave me a way to change what I didn't like about my body, and healthy role models saved me from starving myself and gave me positive results to reach for. Developing healthy mental and physical habits were at least part of the battle.

But when you are a single mom, there isn't much time for work-outs, and then, I took what time I could get and one afternoon a week, my mom watched my daughter so I could spend three hours in the gym. That time was enough to allow my body to build muscle, and to keep my mind sane. For my cardio and fat burning exercise, I had an exercise bike in my two-room apart-ment which I used frequently after my daughter went to bed.

Gaining muscle tipped the scales for me and healthily replaced my bingeing and purging as I added pounds without adding body fat. Developing that exercise discipline was a tedious process that took years for me to make, but one that I believe saved my life. It put control over my body composition into my hands.

There were dangers related to this alternative lifestyle as well that I grew aware of and avoided. I watched at least one friend ruin her life with steroid abuse, which she fell into because of her obsession with managing her diet and her workouts. Even a positive sport or activity can become unhealthy when it becomes your master and takes possession of your mind and body.

SIXTEEN:

Set free

Tired of dead-end jobs and scraping by, I reached for a better future. At that time, nurses were in short supply, and the local college offered full-ride scholarships if you signed a contract to work for them for several years after graduation.

It wasn't my life ambition to be a nurse, but I knew it paid well, so I applied for the program. We would qualify for Medicaid once I quit my job, and that program would help us with food, rent, and medical expenses. I was raised in a proud family, and so the thought of accepting help pained me, but doing it was worth swallowing my pride to get out of poverty. Making a short-term sacrifice for long- term gain was the plan.

That bright future never happened, because one wrong decision on my part landed me with an unexpected pregnancy.

And when I learned of it, there was never any question in my mind of what I was going to do. I was having this baby. Even if I couldn't keep it, I would give the baby life.

It's easy to play out all the "woulda coulda shoulda" scenarios in our minds, but no matter what we might think, there is no way to know what our life would have been if we'd taken a different path or made a different decision at a given moment.

At this point in my life, I married a man (the new babies' father) I didn't love to keep a baby I loved with all of my heart. That was the right decision, despite the difficult circumstances I would find myself in a few years later.

After the baby came, I was a stay-at-home mom of two. I relished my role as wife and mother, and loved everything about staying at home, except having no time to work out. I regained some weight back, and a lack of exercise left me feeling miserable, and it wasn't long until my bingeing and purging started again. Left alone with two children while my husband worked long hours to provide for us created an overwhelming feeling of isolation within me.

The shame of purging, frustrations of carrying baby weight, and being left alone with no one to talk to but a toddler left me depressed. My children made me want to be better, do better, and overcome this debilitating illness, but there was no extra money available for counseling or treatment.

At that time is when I found the book that started me down the road to freedom from purging. You can call this discovery whatever you want, but for me, it was a miracle. My story is not about religion, because I don't want people to judge it on those grounds- it is a chronicle intended to be for anyone, regardless of faith, gender, age, color, or status in life- but I would be remiss if I did not speak the truth about what happened that day.

I came across and read a book on eating disorders entitled "Starving for Attention", which was written by a then-famous figure, Cherry Boone (Pat Boone's daughter). Cherry had suffered for years and nearly died from anorexia nervosa, and when she published her book, it shocked the world.

Descriptions of the abuse she suffered, extreme weight-loss, destructive behaviors, and a skeletal appearance were enough to make readers shudder. And yet, her story was intriguing: in a world of plenty, why would anyone choose to starve their self? It was a good question, and one that millions of Americans were asking. The book unveiled the disease and shattered secrets long hidden by those living behind the anorexic curtain.

I read that book, and then others available on eating disorders, and worked with counselors and kept countless journals, and yet I remained captive to the disease. I wanted to it stop, and I begged God to help me. Still, day after day, the addiction took over.

There was one false belief at the core of my disorder, but I was not yet aware of it. One book revealed the secret that I hid from myself.

I thought I was not worthy of love.

Deep down inside, I believed I had to be perfect in order to be loved.

When you strip away all the layers, all the symptoms, all the unhealthy behaviors, you'd find that the core belief I held was that I had to be perfect to be lovable. Since none of us can ever be perfect, or live up to our own (or other's) ideas of perfection, such a mental requirement puts us in a lose-lose pattern. After a binge-purge episode, I would become overwhelmed by guilt, and following that, self-hatred resulted. No matter how hard I tried or how many promises I made to escape the pattern, the disease won. And, the cycle continued.

Binge, purge, guilt, self-hate. Addiction to anything rolls like that. As humans, we are prone to addictions, but unless you've been there, it is hard to understand the cycle.

Experts now label alcoholism as a disease, along with many forms of self-destructive behaviors that become a lifestyle. Some suggest that the word disease reflects a dis-ease within oneself. At least with my eating disorder, I would say that was true. I lived in dis-ease with myself, my body, my life, my past. But when you are captive to an addiction, it clouds your ability to see clearly or to find a way out of your dis-ease. One of my false beliefs was that when I binged and purged, I was not lovable, and what changed for me one day as I was reading was the realization that God loved me regardless of if I ever changed.

There was a paragraph in one book I read about God loving us just as we are. I don't recall what it said, but I remember the Bible verse quoted.

"But God demonstrates his love own love for us in this: that while we were still sinners, Christ died for us (Romans 5:8)."

That verse told me that there is nothing we can do to earn God's love. NOTHING. Jesus Christ died for me and for you while we were (or are) at our worst.

I pictured myself hanging over the toilet, full of guilt, shame and self-hatred- unworthy, unlovable, disgusting. But I believed in my heart for the first time what that verse said- that God loved me just the same as if I never threw up. And that verse says He loves you the same way. My eating disorder did not make me unworthy of God's love, and stopping it did not make me more worthy of His love. I was worthy of His love just the way I was.

Jesus didn't die for us because we deserved it. He died for us, because he loves us. When we believe Christ was crucified and died for our sins (he paid the ultimate price for us), and nothing we do now or in the future can take that away, it is life-changing. And at the moment I accepted that belief, I underwent a transformation.

I knew in my head that God loved me, but that day, my heart accepted that even if I continued to binge and purge until the day I died, God would love me just the same. He didn't love me because of what I did or didn't do, but just because I existed. He wouldn't love me more if I stopped hanging my head over the toilet and throwing up. And that set me free. In that moment, I knew I would never again make myself throw up.

That was thirty-seven years ago, and to this day, I have not binged or purged.

This does not mean I haven't struggled or felt tempted along the way to return to old habits. It has been quite the opposite. I think if you have an eating disorder long enough (or any addiction), you will deal with it for the rest of your life. I smile when I read accounts by people saying they are free from such-and-such. Not me. I've spent the last thirty-seven years overcoming it, one day at a time, sometimes one thought at a time.

If you think being delivered from bingeing and purging solved all my problems, you would be wrong. At twenty-six years of age, I had two children, and a cheating spouse that verbally and sometimes physically abused us. I was desperately unhappy. The purging had stopped, but my eating disorder remained, and manifested itself in other ways. I would keep myself so busy, I didn't have time to dwell on my unhappy life, and I'd starve myself.

A classic overachiever, I tried to do everything myself. While my husband worked nights and slept days, I managed the children and the house single-handedly. I cleaned, cooked, took care of the yard, homeschooled the children, raised a herd of dairy goats, wrote a book, got my artwork in a local gallery, was active in my church, planted and harvested a garden, canned, and made all our bread from scratch. That list exhausts me reading it, but less than when I was living it.

The decision to starve was deliberate. I remember saying to myself, "I am going to starve myself." It was the only way my sick brain knew how to react to a life that felt out of control. I couldn't control my husband or my life, but I could control my eating. I had stopped purging, but there was still a darkness inside, and it had another weapon of self-destruction. By controlling what I ate, it gave me a false sense of being in control. I also wanted my husband's attention, something he wasn't very good at giving to me.

I started by skipping dinners. I'd eat breakfast and lunch, but little or nothing at dinner. And then I stopped eating sweets, and lunch, and snacks, until I weighed ninety-three pounds. I remember how thin I was, and yet how powerful it felt- like I controlled the world.

I loved my flat stomach, my protruding ribs and bony hips. I enjoyed feeling how tiny my calves felt. Once strong and muscular, my calves, like me, were now gaunt. They had melted away, and I loved it. Maybe it was the endorphins that starving releases like a runner's high that motivated me. Except for gnawing hunger, I felt fantastic! I could wear a size zero jeans. I had arrived at my Utopia and I was the ruler of my kingdom. I decided what I ate, what I didn't and the more weight I lost, the more powerful I felt.

When I was at my thinnest, I got mixed messages from others. Some complimented me and thought I looked great, while others were shocked and concerned. It amazed me that people's perceptions were so different. My face was gaunt, I had almost no body fat, my hip bones protruded, and yet some thought I looked good. But the one person who didn't notice either way was my husband. You would think a spouse would notice or say something about that kind of weight loss. But he didn't.

It was my eye doctor that noticed. After my third eye infection in a short period, he spoke privately to me at an appointment.

"Cynthia, I'm worried about how thin you are. Are you eating?"

"Of course," I said with a smile.

"I think your eye infections are because you aren't eating enough. Your immune system is getting weak. Are you ok?"

I brushed it off with an excuse, but I recall how touched I was that he cared. And I liked the attention.

It shouldn't have been possible to become pregnant as thin as I was, but I did. At first, I lied to myself when I missed my period. It was because I was thin, that's all. I knew for certain when I became deathly ill with morning sickness that I was going to have another baby.

The next three months were the longest of my life. I landed in the hospital several times, unable to stop vomiting. That's the definition of irony: the girl that made herself throw up can't stop herself from throwing up. But this situation was much different. Imagine the worst nausea you've ever had, times five, and that's how I felt every day for months. Once I started throwing up, I'd become dehydrated and would have to be hooked up to IV's in the hospital. The doctor gave me anti-nausea meds, but even those didn't stop it.

The smell of cooking meat, particularly hamburger, was the worst for me. It set off the nausea with uncontrolled vomiting. I never cooked hamburger after the first attack, but my husband did. I would beg him not to, but he did as he pleased, despite my pleas. I'd hide under the covers in the back bedroom, tears running down my face as I wretched over a bowl while he cooked the red meat. Then he'd leave for his evening work shift and leave me alone to deal with my sickness and two children.

When we graduated through several levels of medications that usually helped the nausea, but didn't, my doctor got nervous. The next level of drugs, he said, could be dangerous for the baby. At nine months pregnant, I weighed only 129 pounds. I remember because I stared at the scale, the number burned into my memory, and I thought I was huge and hated getting on the scale.

Somehow, we both survived that pregnancy, and my third child, a healthy girl, although small, was born. She turned out to be the feistiest of all my children. It's no wonder. She had to be a fighter from the start.

Had I not gotten pregnant when I did, I would have kept starving myself. Who knows how far it might have gone? My children gave me a reason to live and I am grateful for them. It was because of them I stayed in my marriage for eight years, and also why I eventually left it.

Our home was peaceful when my husband was gone, but it was miserable when he was around. He was angry most of the time, and he took it out on us. The children suffered the most from it, and no amount of begging, pleading or threatening convinced him we needed help. Even the cat fled his presence and would hide under the stairwell and hiss.

I kneeled before him one day, begging for us to seek help. His words still ring in my ears.

"I've been this way my whole life and I'm probably never going to change."

At least he spoke his truth. I got up off my knees, wiped away my tears, and accepted it. Live with it or leave. Those were my choices.

I hadn't worked for eight years, and had few employable skills, but I was determined to get me and my children out of the situation. The only thing I regretted after we fled was that I hadn't done it sooner. By then, dysfunction had done much damage to each of us. I wish I could say our family lived happily ever after, but we didn't. For me, leaving was the beginning of a long struggle to raise my children. It would be years before we thrived, but no matter how hard leaving was, it was the right choice for us. To stay would have been worse.

We all make decisions we think are right at the time. It may be years later before we know if that decision was a good choice, but at the time, it was what seemed right. If only life came with a road map that you could view before you decided which path to take. I repeated many of the same mistakes my mom and her mom made, ones I swore I wouldn't make, thinking somehow, I was better than them. I judged my mom harshly until I realized she did the best she could in her life. She, too, was a victim until she decided not to be. And she has become a great example of love, forgiveness, and freedom to me.

My oldest brother Jeff and I are now good friends. After his twenty-year marriage fell apart, I was there to support him. I'd been through what he was experiencing, so I understood his pain and frustration. I would call him, make him laugh, and encourage him that life would get better. Since he had gone through a divorce, he could understand me and now we both belonged to the same club.

We became friends, sitting back-to-back under a tree at an event for my oldest daughter. She was running in a mud race, and we both came to watch. My brother traveled hundreds of miles to watch the race and spend some time with us. While we waited for her to appear among the runners, we had one of the best conversations in our life. He humbly apologized for his part in hurting me when we were growing up. And I understood he was also a victim of my dad's lack of character.

As the oldest and a boy, I felt he suffered the most when we were young. He carried the burden of looking out for all three of us and had to bear an enormous weight on his shoulders well before he was ready to handle it. He rose to the challenge then, doing the best he could. I admire, respect and love my big brother more than I can say. And I'm so glad we had the chance to mend our fences under a pine tree in the forest.

My brothers were good looking, athletic, outdoorsy, and hard-working- boys that any father would be proud of. It must have been hard for them to be left behind, discarded like trash, as the new baby boy got all of their father's attention. It was hard on all of us, and it wasn't fair.

Life isn't fair, though, and no amount of wishing or hoping will make it so. But there is always a choice in how we handle it: remain the victim, or rise above it.

Hopefully, each generation rises above the previous one, improving their lives and their children's lives. We live in a broken world and, to some extent, we are all broken. Putting pieces back together takes time, patience, and perseverance. It is a process for which there is no shortcut. The first step towards healing is a desire to become whole again. No matter where you are on your journey, you can decide to get help and mend the brokenness. You are not alone. Many struggle with eating disorders. Many people you see everyday deal with an eating disorder.

They don't wear a sign around their necks or a T-shirt that says, "Ask me about my eating disorder", though. Too many suffer in silence or hopelessness. But many others have over-come the disorder and gone on to happy lives. It all starts with a single step.

I am no longer a victim, but instead, I am the leading lady of my life, and you can be the leading man or lady of your own life as well. I have traveled on from my past to enjoy a successful career, buy two houses by myself, and have never returned to starving, bingeing, or purging. My life has been an arduous journey, but I gained wisdom along the path to recovery- wisdom that I share with you in the next section of this book. The road to my recovery was rocky, but it made me who I am today- a happy, healthy woman who loves her life.

If we could wave a magic wand, to be free of what ails us, it would be so much simpler, but we would miss out on the dance of life, and in that dance is where the magic is.

"Everyone wants to live on top of the mountain, but all the happiness and growth occurs while you are climbing it." ~Andy Rooney

You may not believe that happiness will ever find you, or that you will recover, but I can tell you from experience that amid the chaos and the struggle, happiness is waiting to happen. The hardest times I experienced were the times of my greatest growth, which led to my greatest happiness.

While I thought I'd seen the hardest times in my life while raising my children, I was wrong. Little did I know that my eating disorder would manifest itself in a life-threatening way years later, and I would have no control over it. Instead of me starving myself, my body tried to starve itself because of more deep emotional pain. It was a long road to hell and back before I arrived at the door of happiness. Those were dark days, as death knocked on my door.

That's another story though, which I tell in my book "Happiness Came With a Cat" (New Edition). If you'd like to find out how my eating disorder, along with Seasonal Affective Disorder (SAD), grief, and depression almost took my life until I finally found happiness, check it out on Amazon (available in Kindle or paperback) or on my website at CynthiaStarBooks. com/Adult-genre

After I wrote the happiness book, it gave me the strength to write this one. It is difficult to be honest and to share such personal details, but I do because I believe my stories will touch many lives and help others. I hope this book helps you or someone that you love. If it does, I'd love to hear about it.

Send me an email at cynastar019@gmail.com if you care to share about it.

A deeper understanding of eating disorders has led to more sophisticated treatment methods. Programs that address the source of the eating disorder and help families to work together and to heal are available. Do not suffer in silence. Reach out for help, and don't stop until you find it.

The purpose of the remaining chapters in this book is to share lessons that I learned on my road to recovery, and provide you with hope that you, too, can achieve freedom. If you are a family member or a loved one related to the sufferer, the disorder also affects you. I encourage you to go through these lessons as well.

You can work through them together as a family, or complete them with a friend, with a counselor, or by yourself. The wisdom I've gained and the coping mechanisms I still use to manage this disorder may help you or someone else you know who needs them. Isn't that why you picked up this book?

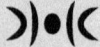

PART TWO

Recovery Lessons

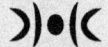

I'm not a therapist. These Recovery Lessons are intended to supplement your treatment with a professional, not replace it. I strongly recommend that you find a good therapist or psychiatrist, and maybe seeking family treatment would also be helpful, depending on the severity of the disorder. There are many options available, and I encourage you to seek the right one for you.

Whether you are the person with an eating disorder, or are a family member, friend, spouse or partner to that person, you need support for yourself and help to understand the disease. You may play a part in the dysfunction and not know it- but you are affected by it, so seek help in this journey, by yourself or with your loved one. Even if you get help alone, I still encourage you to do so.

It can be devastating to watch someone struggle with an eating disorder. Early detection and treatment increase the chances for their recovery, so consider getting professional help as early as possible.

I've included space in this book for you to write answers to questions or reflections on concepts throughout each lesson. You may use the space provided here or start a journal or notebook of your own. You might call it My Recovery Journal or come up with another title yourself. If you are reading the Kindle version, you may find that one of the new apps for journaling works well for you. They offer privacy with the use of a password and some offer writing prompts daily or weekly.

It is imperative in recovery work to get your thoughts out of your head and onto paper or some sort of journal.

If you are not the person with the eating disorder but are close to them, I would encourage you to also keep a journal. It will help you to recognize patterns of behavior, both in yourself and in your loved one. It is usually the person with the eating disorder that gets the most treatment, but those close to him or her suffer also, and so I encourage you to take your own journey through these recovery pages. You may recognize yourself in some of these lessons, and, who knows, you might benefit from completing some of these exercises.

At first, it might be difficult to write your thoughts or feelings down, and that's ok. Be gentle with yourself. Start with just one reflection or answer as you go along. Even if your answers are one-word answers, that is progress.

There is no expectation that you work through the lessons in order, or that you answer all the questions. I've included many questions for each lesson, but you don't have to answer all of them. Some you may find helpful, and others redundant. This is your journey, and you get to set the pace at which you work. I want you to work through the lessons as you wish, skipping around, coming back, years or months later. Remember, recovery is a process, so allow yourself time to work through things without making it a pass or fail exercise. You decide what lessons to focus on and how long to take on any lesson.

It is up to you if you wish to share your answers with a counselor, friend, or your family. You may find it helpful to discuss the lessons or your answers with someone you trust, and I encourage you to do so when you feel comfortable.

An eating disorder is like an onion, it has layers. You peel back one layer, only to find another one. When you look at a whole onion, you don't see the layers. You would never know they were there until you peel it. And you can't see the next layer until you peel back the first one. It might take years to peel back the layers of your eating disorder. That's ok, because it took years to create those layers. The goal is to recognize the next layer when it reveals itself, so that you can peel it away and not judge yourself because you found another layer.

If you binge eat or often eat too much, you should know besides emotional layers, **there are biological factors built into our brains that encourage us to overeat.** You are not only fighting the addiction cycle, but a survival mechanism designed to keep you overeating. Understanding this may help in your recovery. There are various articles available online if you care to read more about the findings of such experiments. Once such experiment is cited below:

"In lab experiments, Thomas Kash, PhD, the John R. Andrews Distinguished Professor in the Department of Pharmacology at the University of North Carolina School of Medicine, and his colleagues discovered a specific network of cellular communication emanating from the emotion-processing region of the brain, motivating mice to keep eating tasty food even though their basic energy needs had been met."

Kash is a member of the UNC Bowles Center for Alcohol Studies

Article published April 24, 2019

If you care to read the article, it can be found online at: UNC Health and UNC School of Medicine newsroom. It is no simple task to overcome an eating disorder, no matter what that disorder might be. So be patient with yourself.

RECOVERY LESSON #1:

Get creative

> "Our dreams may seem impossible, but our creativity
> can turn them into reality."
> ~*Malala Yousafzai*

What does creativity have to do with fighting an eating dis-order? Everything. Look around you. Everything you see is a creation of someone. This book, your cup, that car. The clothes you wear, the food you eat, the table you set. Creativity exists in the universe and in our physical world.

Creativity is an expression that comes from our soul. And I believe it has the power to heal a person from the inside out. You might think you are not creative, but I believe creativity is intrinsic in all of us. Making music, dancing, drawing, painting, rhyming, sketching, throwing pottery, cooking, even coloring is being creative. The list is endless.

Depression, grief, anger, sadness, and even boredom can strip away our creative nature. But it remains there, buried beneath the layers of your eating disorder. Your job is to discover it again. Creativity releases the child in us. It requires us to use our imagination, and gets us outside of ourselves and in touch with fun. The more creative you let yourself be, the happier and healthier you become. It may take time for you to get in touch with your creativity, but that is ok.

Do you recall coloring as a child?

Or tracing your hand to make a Thanksgiving turkey?

Maybe you enjoyed making a snowman out of cotton balls or had fun dipping your brush in watercolors and spreading hues across a page?

The goal of this lesson is to encourage you to reconnect with your childlike creativity and to find some unfettered fun.

For example, I like to paint rocks. I am a self-published author of 10 books, and have had my art displayed in a gallery, but I like to paint rocks. I use silly, fun, simple designs and have no rules attached to my process, except that I have fun creating pretty rocks. I call it "Rock Therapy".

I'm not even very good at it, but I give myself permission to do it anyway. I give away my rocks, usually to strangers, by leaving them randomly along the trails where I hike. The idea started when I was out hiking and found a hand-painted rock tucked beneath a bush that someone else left there for others to find. Do I pick it up or leave it there?

I left it, but when I returned to that place the next week, the rock was gone. That made me smile, as I imagined the person taking the time to hand paint the rock leaving it for others to have with no strings attached. The rock seemed to say, take me or leave me- you decide.

I wondered who took the rock. The colorful stone must have motivated someone to pick it up, and I assume they took it home. And that reflection sparked my creativity to do the same- to bless others with gifts of my creative rocks. I've left many of them along trails, and they always disappear.

I like to think my rock meant something to the person who picked it up and put it in their pocket. Maybe it inspired them, moved them, or made them think of someone else to whom they gave the rock. The possibilities of why they took the rock with them are endless, and considering them is part of the fun in my exercise.

No matter how silly it may seem, practicing creativity on any level is healing. It helps us to express emotions that words can't express, especially if we have a hard time talking about something. Even if it's expressing what we consider a negative emotion, being creative is an outlet of our inner selves.

I lost touch with my creative side during a tough time in my life. It took some work for me to get it back. To spur my creativity,

I made a "Creative Date" with myself once a week. I set aside an hour or two every week for creative adventures.

My first adventure took me outside on a warm spring day. There was a path close to our house that led to a creek close by our house with grass along its bank. I lay on the soft carpet, gazing up, trying to find pictures in the clouds like I'd done as a child. For the longest time, all I saw were clouds moving in the sky. But then… they came alive before my eyes. The image I most remembered was a majestic horse, neck bowed, muscles bulging, wings spread wide as he flew above. It was burned in my imagination and I raced home to draw the horse.

On my next creative date, I took myself down to the local skateboard park. I was driven to get that horse out of my head and onto the concrete. With a bucket of colored chalk, the sketch I'd made, and an endless concrete canvas, a life-sized equine appeared. The skateboarders looked on, asking questions as I worked, wondering who this crazy lady was that was invading their territory. But when I finished, they gathered around my horse and thanked me for sharing it with them.

They were laughing, skating around, and through the bright colored horse as I left. I had fun; they had fun; and we shared a connection through a chalk horse that melted away in a day. The sillier it seems, the more fun you will have. Allow yourself freedom of expression to go with what delights you. The lesson here is to unleash your creativity, and there are no rules.

Why not set a creative date with yourself? One day a week, allot time for an adventure. Visit a museum, an art gallery, a local shop or lie beneath the clouds on a spring day.

Buy a coloring book, a sketch pad, or gather rocks. Dust off your imagination and get inspired. You decide what might spur your creativity.

Look around for inspiration and ask the child inside, what would delight them?

There is a good reason I started with creativity in your first lesson. Because being creative can help you get in touch with and express your innermost feelings- the ones you can't talk about or share; the ones you don't know exist or you may have lost touch with.

In many of the following lessons, I suggest ways you can use creativity to express yourself. There may be thoughts, feelings, or emotions that are buried deep in your soul that, by expressing them creatively, can help you get in touch with what is eating at you.

I encourage you to try some of the creative activities I've suggested, or come up with some of your own. The more freedom of expression you allow yourself, the better. You get to decide what that looks like, feels like, or sounds like. Ready to get creative?

RECOVERY LESSON #2:

False beliefs

> "There is only one cause of unhappiness: The false beliefs you have in your head, beliefs so widespread, so commonly held, that it never occurs to you to question them."
> *~ Anthony de Mello~*

My false beliefs came from me. I viewed my heavenly Father like I saw my earthly dad, and I believed I had to earn His love by how I looked, or based on what I did or didn't do. What I realized the day that I was set free from my purging addiction was God's unconditional love for me. Even if I died living in my worst condition, God still loved me fully as if I had never had an addiction. There was absolutely nothing I could do to earn His love, or to lose it. All I had to do was to believe that truth and accept it. Doing that changed my life.

I am not here to preach the Bible or teach religion. I am only here to tell you what changed my life's direction. What I do hope will happen is that you will believe you can overcome your own eating disorder. With or without a miracle, what I learned over the years can help set you free- not just from an eating disorder, but from drugs, sex, alcohol, or whatever else holds you captive.

Recovery is a road less traveled, and along the way, you will encounter speed bumps, curves, and stop signs. There may be times you total your vehicle (your body, your life, your future) and you have to start again. The only thing that matters is that you learn from your experience and start your engine again. As long as you draw breath, as long as your spirit remains in your body, there is hope.

The first question I want you to ask yourself is:

"What false beliefs am I holding onto?"

_____

_____

Only you know the answer. And it might take a lot of time to dig through all the layers to find it. Keep asking yourself (and maybe others around you) that question until you know you found the answer. You might even have several answers, that's ok.

Here are some questions to help prompt you in this exercise.

Control: We cannot control the actions of others, only our own actions and reactions. Eating disorders are often about control and they can create a false sense of control.

Does my life feel out of control?

_____

If yes, why?

_____

What makes me feel in control?

_____

What makes me feel out of control?

_____

What behaviors might I be exhibiting that give me a false sense of control?

_____

Do I try to control others?

_____

How are they affected by my desire to be in control?

_____

What would happen if I let go of that control?

_____

_____

Do I feel controlled by others?

_____

If yes, who do I feel controls me?

_____

What words or actions from others make me feel controlled?

_____

_____

_____

You could do an art project to express how control feels to you.

Write your ideas below.

What does control look like?

_____

What does it look like for you to be out of control?

_____

Example: I did an art project when I was working with my counselor. I felt great relief over a positive decision I made for my emotional health, so she asked me what relief looks like to me.

At first, I was unsure where to begin. She had me close my eyes, breathe deeply, and think about what relief felt like in my body. Then she asked me to think about what that would look like on paper. I grabbed a pad of brightly colored construction paper, a glue stick, and my imagination. I tore pieces of colored paper in various sizes and shapes that represented a rainbow. Then I took a blue piece of paper, tore some green for grass along the bottom and glued it in place. I arranged the colored pieces in the shape of a rainbow on my blue-sky page.

Finally, I tore a jagged round piece representing the sun. Tearing the pieces, gluing them on the page, and allowing my feelings to appear on the page was delightful, even though I completed the project in about ten minutes. I let myself be free to express what I couldn't say with words.

Try this exercise with control or any emotion you want to explore a bit deeper. You can choose any medium you want. Or even use a musical instrument.

Ask yourself:

What does the emotion I'm feeling look like to me? Example: control or lack of control.

_____

What does it sound like?

_____

What does it feel like?

_____

Perfectionism: No one is perfect. We all make mistakes. We often think if we looked this way or that way, then we would be happy. The desire to be perfect often manifests itself in an eating disorder. It starts with the false belief that you must be perfect to be loved, accepted, or feel good about yourself. I shared with you my thoughts on perfection, where they came from, and how I developed them. It took me years to realize that perfectionism was one of the false beliefs that I was holding onto. It may take you years as well.

Here are some questions you can ask yourself:

Do I feel lovable only if I'm perfect?

_____

Why?

_____

_____

What is my idea of perfection?

_____

_____

Where did my perfectionism come from?

_____

_____

What would happen if I wasn't perfect?

_____

_____

How would it feel like to be loved simply for existing?

_____

_____

_____

What if I loved myself just because I exist?

_____

_____

Who do I love even though I know they aren't perfect?

_____

Would I love them more if they were perfect?

_____

Why or why not?

_____

_____

_____

There is no judgement in your answers. Just let them be what they want to be.

Sit with your answers for a while. You can come back to this exercise as many times as you want. Some days, your answers may be different. That's ok.

RECOVERY LESSON #3:

Learning is winning

> "I never lose. I either win or I learn."
> ~ *Nelson Mandela*

Black or white. Yes or no. All or nothing. These pairs express opposites, definitive and concrete. I lived in this kind of world in my mind, filled with dualities with little to no grays in between.

We need boundaries in our lives to protect ourselves and to keep us in check, but when we live inside of strict lines that we have set up for ourselves, life closes in on us pretty fast. Perfectionism lives inside the lines, and perfectionists believe that to go outside of the lines is death (physical or mental). We see life as win or lose.

What Nelson Mandela says in the above quote is that he made life experiences a win-win. Even if you choose a course that causes you to take a step back, or to fall short, you don't lose. You win, as long as you learn something. I call these steps "opportunities to learn." All I know is, I have given myself lots of opportunities to learn. I once asked a friend how many more *opportunities* I had to experience related to a particular circumstance. She said, "As many as you need until you learn the lesson."

In my head, I was always "either" … Either good or bad, right or wrong, fat or thin. And I beat myself up verbally if I was on the wrong side of the line I'd drawn. Life has lots of black and white. Scientific rules like gravity are undeniable. But life, I've learned, also has a lot of gray areas. Learning to live in the gray areas leads to recovery.

Remember that I said an eating disorder is about lies that you tell yourself until you believe them? If you had a friend that kept lying to you, would you continue to be their friend? How many times would you let them lie to you before you confronted the problem or stopped hanging around them? Likewise, you have to stop believing your own lies.

You must distrust the things you tell yourself until you prove you can trust yourself (which may be never). Until then, you will need to have a counselor, friend, or family member to help guide you in setting healthy expectations for yourself- someone emotionally healthy that you respect and trust, in the way I respected my counselor when she said I wasn't allowed to weigh less than one-hundred pounds. She drew a line in the sand for me, and because I trusted and respected her, I followed it.

Don't trust yourself, or anyone else with an eating disorder, or someone who manipulates, controls or demeans you for guidance or therapy. Seek help from a mentor, a counselor, or respected person you admire, and ask them to help you sift the truth from the lies that you tell yourself, and seek advice from them about any big life or relationship decisions you face.

Your friends, spouse, or family members should not be your therapist. They can support you, guide you, and encourage you, but they should not be your therapist.

There are differences among counselors and therapists in terms of their abilities and effectiveness. Some will ask you the tough questions you won't ask yourself. Others will let you spend hours talking about your feelings without helping you to see any errors in your thinking or offering you any concrete help for your recovery. Run from the latter type, and go find yet another one. There are plenty of good counselors and therapists out there. I've gone through my share, and I will find one again if I feel the need.

A good counselor listens, guides you to see the truth for yourself, asks you tough questions at the right time, and develops a recovery plan with you. How far down the eating disorder path you have traveled determines how screwed up your thinking has become and the level of help you need. You will need therapy and guidance, maybe for the rest of your life. But let that be okay.

Through the years, I have had friends I've gone to for guidance. Not for therapy, but for guidance with thought patterns and decisions. Realizing that my thinking was skewed, I acknowledged that I needed guidance. When you don't know how to think in healthy ways, until you do, seek help. You will need both guidance and therapy.

It also took me years to learn that how I define success or failure is where some magic for recovery lies. Although she doesn't know it, a friend helped me to see how extreme my thinking about failure was, because I remember her reaction to my reaction to an incident vividly.

We were rehearsing a program that our Rotary Club would perform for the public as a fundraiser. Without realizing it, I said something that offended another Rotarian in front of everyone. Since I was the club president, when I realized my error, I felt I should know better and took it as a personal failure. I lashed out at myself verbally, and by the time my friend found me, I was crying. When I explained what had happened, she smiled and gave me a hug.

"So what? You made a mistake. It's not the end of the world."

My face was blank. I didn't understand her flippancy. It was the end of the world to me. I messed up, I failed, I deserve punishment.

"Did you apologize?" She asked.

"Yes, several times."

"Then let it go and move on," she said. "Come on, let's go join everyone."

My mind could not comprehend someone could handle a situation so easily, because I only knew one way, which was to take things personally, feel like a failure, and beat myself up. A new day dawned for me when I realized she was right. I played her words over in my head until I let the situation go, and used her method the next time I felt like a failure.

My friend taught me a valuable lesson. Just because I make a mistake doesn't mean I'm a failure. So, I messed up- everyone does. I just need to take responsibility for my actions and move on. I had to give myself permission to fail and believe it would not define my success. I still use this mental exercise. After all these years, I still start to berate myself. The difference is, I recognize my self-destructive behavior and now stop myself.

My friend did not judge me. She was gentle and understanding. I judged myself much more harshly than anyone else had. What if I stopped judging myself and accepted it for what it was? A mistake.

Now, in the same situation, I would tell myself, "I made a mistake, but I am not a failure."

A healthy mindset is one that allows for gray areas. If we learn, we win. That all-or-nothing thinking will keep you locked in an eating disorder.

Example:

When I was attending college, I strove for perfection. In my mind, I had to make the Dean's list, or I was a failure. Even if it cost me my health, caused overwhelming stress, and filled me with unhappiness, I pushed for a GPA above 3.5. My pursuit of perfection in school pushed me over the edge and led me to drop out. Was that worth it? The cost of perfection was expensive.

What if instead of making all A's, I let myself get B's or C's? What a difference that might have made. I would have been much happier and balanced, and able to continue in my studies. I might have taken more writing classes and pursued a career that worked with my strengths. Perhaps I would have become a journalist or worked for a magazine, writing articles and traveling the country.

All the "woulda coulda, shoulda"s in the world will not change my past. But I can take the lessons learned along the way and apply them to the present. This chapter's painful lesson reminds me that chasing perfection comes at a high cost.

Now, I ask myself, "What if you didn't have to be perfect? What would that look like?"

Example of a recent conversation in my head:

"There isn't enough time to do a workout. I need at least an hour for a worthwhile workout. I guess I won't work out at all." That's the old me talking.

The new me recognized my all-or-nothing thinking, and talked back.

"You have twenty minutes. Doing a short workout is better than having no workout at all."

I took the time I had, did a short workout, and felt better.

I told myself, "Good job! You took advantage of what time you had."

The old me would have said, after forfeiting my one-hour workout, "You missed your workout. You are lazy and worthless. Now you have to work out for two hours."

At first, you may need help to see the hard lines you've drawn in your life. With practice, you will catch yourself facing them and can use self-talk to get past them.

Identify small opportunities where you can introduce compromises, like I did in my example of the workout. You can apply this exercise to your eating habits too.

Example of all-or-nothing thinking:

"I ate a cookie (or two cookies or a piece of cake or?). I'm a failure. I might as well eat all of them."

"I binged so I'm a failure. I might as well keep bingeing."

"I threw up today. I'm worthless and I'll never stop. I might as well throw this food up also."

Replace those thoughts with things like:

"I ate this cookie/cake/pizza. That's ok. It's just a cookie/cake/piece. I'm making progress."

Or:

"I did better than yesterday. It's ok to eat some, but I don't need to eat it all."

Come up with your own replacement statements. Pay attention to your black-and-white and all-or-nothing thinking. Note when and where it happens and why you think you enter that mode then. Come up with positive affirmations to tell yourself to replace the negative words in your usual thoughts.

Soon, gentler thinking will become a habit and you will see larger areas of your life that might need more gray and less black and white.

Questions to ask:

Do I allow for gray areas in my life?

What would it look like if I did?

_____

_____

_____

What are some of my black-and-white beliefs?

_____

_____

_____

Think of a time where you applied black-and-white/good-or-bad/all-or-nothing thinking to a situation and write about it.

_____

_____

_____

In the situation you just described, how did you feel after?

_____

_____

_____

If in your mind you failed, how did that feel?

_____

_____

_____

If in your mind you succeeded, how did that feel?

_____

_____

_____

Is there anything that you might have done that would have felt better?

_____

_____

_____

What things did you say to yourself about how you reacted in that situation?

_____

_____

_____

What are some positive things you could say to yourself about the situation?

_____

_____

_____

RECOVERY LESSON #4:

Be your own best friend

)|●|(

"The greatest gift you can give yourself is the gift of
self-love. Be your own best friend."

~Unknown

Have you ever had a best friend? How do you treat them?

Well, I hope very well, if you want to keep them as a friend.
That is what I had to learn to do- to treat myself like I would
my best friend. At first, I wasn't a wonderful friend to myself,
but with time and practice, I got better at it.

The first step I took to be a better friend to myself was to talk
kinder to myself, something I appreciated experiencing from
my friends.

If I catch myself saying mean, negative, or derogatory things to myself, I ask myself, *would I say this to my best friend?* Then why would I treat myself this way?

Pay attention to how you treat yourself. Are you saying positive or negative things to yourself?

Write at least five things you said to yourself in the last twenty-four hours.

_____

_____

_____

_____

_____

Were they positive or negative?

_____

Erase or cross out the negative ones.

Highlight the positive things. Repeat those words to yourself as many times as it takes to feel better. If you feel bad again, repeat the positive affirmations until you let the bad feelings go.

I still have to do this exercise, sometimes daily. I'm so hard on myself that I relive situations where I think I screwed up, but now I imagine a friend doing what I did, and think of what I would say to her or him in the situation. Would I want my friend to keep beating themselves up over this?

Then why do I keep beating myself up?

What would my best friend would tell me about this situation?

_____

_____

_____

_____

Friends often give us gifts. It may be a gift of their time, talents, or something they think we would enjoy. One thing I did recently for a few of my friends was to get out several personal gifts I'd spent months gathering, wrapped each of them, and then mailed them to those friends. Several had traveled a long way to attend my wedding, and each gave me the gifts of their time and love. My way of showing how much I appreciated their friendships was to send them gifts with a nice card.

What are some gifts you could give to yourself?

_____

_____

_____

Pick at least one thing on the list and gift it to yourself. You could even mail yourself a gift.

How did that gift make you feel?

_____

_____

_____

Why did you pick that gift for yourself?

_____

_____

_____

Write yourself a friendly note and say the things that a dear friend might tell you. I know you think this is silly, but if you did as many nice things for yourself that you do for your friends, you might start to like yourself.

Maybe giving yourself time to doing something you really enjoy would make you smile?

Ask yourself what you would really like to do if you allowed yourself the time.

_____

_____

Draw? Paint? Color?

_____

Take a walk or go for a hike?

_____

Share time with a friend?

_____

Relax in bubble bath surrounded by candles?

_____

What guilty pleasure do you deny yourself because you don't think you deserve it? And I do not mean something you think you have to do, but some activity that would be enjoyable for you.

_____

_____

_____

Plan at least an hour this week for the activity and put it on your calendar. Then write about how it felt to allow yourself to do the one thing you really wanted to do.

_____

_____

_____

_____

What if you allowed yourself an hour a week, every week, for this activity?

_____

_____

_____

_____

What would it feel like to make time for doing the one thing you really want to do?

_____

_____

_____

_____

Is there something you've always wanted? Even something silly or fun that you wouldn't normally buy for yourself?

_____

_____

_____

_____

Maybe guitar lessons?

_____

What about an art or dance class?

_____

A special pen? Or a lovely smelling candle?

_____

Time by yourself?

_____

_____

_____

_____

Write some ideas and pick at least one gift to give yourself.

_____

_____

_____

How does it feel to give yourself gifts?

_____

_____

_____

How does it feel when you give gifts to your friend/s?

_____

_____

_____

Did it feel as good to gift yourself as it did when you give someone else a gift?

_____

Why or why not?

_____

_____

_____

_____

When you have a best friend, what is the first thing you want to do when anything exciting, sad, or interesting happens?

You want to tell them.

I have a friend that enjoys every detail of my stories. When I try to make a long story short, she stops me and says, "No, go back. I want to hear this."

A good friend listens. Maybe not every friend loves the details so much as my friend, but they want to hear what you have to say. To be a good friend to yourself, you need to say what you think and feel- and listen to yourself. Talk about what is happening in your life to yourself. A journal is the perfect place to do that.

Getting feelings out, especially on paper, is very healing. Looking back on what I wrote a day, a week, or a year ago is enlightening. Reading my own thoughts of where I was at that moment also helps me to understand myself better. And it will help you too.

A genuine friend will be honest, but kind with their words. They will talk you into things that are good for you and out of the things that might be harmful. Learning to be honest with myself was a huge part of my recovery, because if I can't be honest with myself, how can I ever hope to be honest with anyone else?

If I'm writing in a journal, and I say things that might hurt someone if they read it, I shred the pages afterwards, so no one ever finds it. But I let my feelings out.

There may be thoughts and feelings I don't know I'm holding inside until they reveal themselves. That's ok. The healthier I get emotionally and physically, the more I recognize such things. And so will you.

I do allow myself to say what I really feel now- maybe not to others, but to myself, out loud, in my journal, or in my head. I might cuss, scream, cry, or yell, but I do whatever it takes to get those thoughts and feelings out.

What do you really want to say?

_____

_____

_____

_____

_____

_____

_____

_____

_____

_____

What is eating you inside that you need to let out?

_____

_____

_____

_____

_____

_____

What would those feelings look like?

_____

_____

_____

What do they sound like?

_____

_____

_____

Is there anything else you could do to express those feelings?

_____

_____

_____

_____

What about writing a poem or a song about it?

_____

_____

_____

_____

_____

_____

You could make puzzle pieces out of cardboard or construction paper.

_____

_____

_____

What about making yourself a friendship bracelet- maybe one for each arm?

_____

_____

_____

You are allowed to have your feelings. We can't always say what we think or feel to others because it might be emotionally harmful to them, or you might be afraid to say what you really feel. But you are allowed to feel those things. You can write those thoughts and feelings down, and then shred the paper.

You can shout them out if you're alone or outside. You can tell your counselor about them. You can call a trusted friend or a family member.

You could write a story or act them out in a play.

You could make a puppet and let the puppet express your feelings (this might be really fun!).

But getting our feelings out in a healthy way is allowed- and necessary.

Pretend your best friend is telling you the same feelings you would like to express. If he or she had an eating disorder, how would you talk to them?

_____

_____

_____

_____

_____

_____

_____

_____

_____

_____

_____

Would you berate them for having those feelings?

Would you judge them harshly and verbally abuse them? No, you wouldn't.

Then stop doing those things to yourself.

Think about what friends do for one another. What things do you wish a friend might do for you? Imagine being your own best friend and what that looks like, sounds like, and feels like. Treat yourself with love, instead of judgment, the way you would a best friend.

Here's an exercise to try:

Write down ten things you like about yourself. Post them some place you can see them. On your wall calendar, in your car, on your desk, on your mirror, or on your wall. Now you can use those as affirmations when you need them.

Here is a self-reflection I had while writing this chapter.

This chapter was one of the hardest for me to write. I struggled with what to say and how to say it, often feeling frustrated and stuck. I avoided writing it numerous times, wanting to skip it because it was challenging for me to write.

It was a hard chapter to write because I realized this is an area where I need to do more work on myself, being my best friend. And that realization surprised me. Instead of judging myself for it, though, I admitted it to myself- and to you, my reader- and that, my friend, is, for me, taking a step forward.

There will be surprises on your recovery journey- areas that you think you've conquered that return to visit and say, "I'm still here." That is ok, because now you are aware of them, and you can work on them, being kinder to yourself as you do with your beloved friend. You.

RECOVERY LESSON #5:

Self-talk

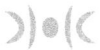

> "Have you realized that most of your unhappiness in life is due to the fact that you are listening to yourself instead of talking to yourself?"
> ~*Martyn Lloyd Jones*

The awful things I said to myself were the reason I developed and stayed in my eating disorder, because I believed what I was telling myself. Talking to myself was also the way I found freedom. By talking myself into good things (thoughts) and out of bad ones, I was able to overcome bad habits in positive ways. This is the single biggest lesson I learned in my recovery: talk positively to yourself. I still use this skill every day.

Being a friend to yourself, talking to yourself in a friendly manner, and using self-talk are interconnected. Once you become your own best friend, it will be much easier to use positive self-talk.

I turn things to positive when I catch myself saying things like:

"You're an idiot."

"You are worthless."

"You are fat."

You are what you think, and believe it or not, you can learn to control your thought patterns. All of those thoughts are going around in your head, anyway. Why not use them to help you, instead of hurt you?

Start writing down the negative things you say to yourself. Keep track of them for a day or two. I think it will surprise you how many times a day you say mean things to yourself.

Would you stay friends with someone who said such mean things all the time? Would you say those mean things to your friends? They probably wouldn't be your friends very long if you did. If you wouldn't treat others that way, why do you allow yourself to talk to you like that?

Now write down at least ten positive things you can say about yourself, and memorize them, so that you can have them on the tip of your tongue.

_____

_____

_____

_____

_____

_____

_____

_____

_____

_____

Having trouble? Think about what you would you say to a friend that was struggling with this?

Listening for negative self-talk and turning it into positive talk is a huge key to recovery. **If you get nothing else out of this book, this lesson alone will change your life.**

You'll get good at catching yourself in mid-sentence and turning those thoughts around. It takes practice, but the first step is to realize what you are doing.

Now, when I hear myself say, "You're an idiot", I stop myself and say, "You are smart. You just did something stupid, but you are not stupid."

If I'm alone, I say it out loud to myself. Then I smile because I know how powerful that one act is. The longer you have been using negative self-talk, the harder it is to turn it into something positive. But every time you do, you take a step forward.

Using self-talk to say positive things to yourself is one part of this exercise. Using self-talk to talk yourself through uncomfortable situations is the other.

I started using self-talk to get over the feeling of a full stomach. I equated having a full stomach with being fat. If I felt full, I feared I was going to get fat. People without an eating disorder don't have a clue about the struggle we go through after we eat when we are used to having an empty stomach. When having an empty stomach is the norm for you, it will take some work to get used to a full stomach, or even one with some food in there. With time, feeling full will become the norm, but until it does, you will need to talk yourself through to it.

First, I had to talk myself through having some food in my stomach. Later, I had to tell myself having a full stomach felt comfortable and normal. But enabling this change took a lot of work during those first few meals. The transition from feeling no food to some food within is uncomfortable, just as having an empty stomach once felt uncomfortable. Are you willing to be uncomfortable to become comfortable? Transitioning between the two conditions is most uncomfortable because you're used to the old way (having an empty stomach), and it will feel icky until you spend some time in the new space (having food in your stomach), until the feeling of having food in your stomach becomes your new norm. Then, and only then, will it feel comfortable.

Doing anything new feels uncomfortable at first. Starting a new job, making a new friend, or learning something for the first time all initially feel awkward. But after weeks, days, or months, what felt uncomfortable becomes comfortable and your new norm. It's the space between leaving the old and starting the new that causes us discomfort. It helps for you to recognize this position. When part of you, either physically or mentally, is still living in the old, you're not fully in the new and it causes discomfort.

We wish for things the way they were because we were used to that. Even when the new is better, brighter, or may improve our lives, it is human nature to cling to what we know, to travel the course of least resistance.

Change is hard for us. We like routine and prefer well-worn pathways. Our minds forget that, at one time, what is now comfortable for us was once uncomfortable. Recognizing when you are in transition will allow you to get to a better place. When you don't recognize the transitional feeling, being uncomfortable may drive you back to old habits. But when you are aware of the transitional space, you can choose to walk and work through it, a little at a time. Self-talk is a powerful tool to help get you through a transitional space. When used in a positive manner, it will help you overcome an eating disorder.

If you are anorexic, it may be hard for you to have food in your stomach. If you are bulimic, it may be hard for you not to purge. Envision yourself feeling happy and content after a meal, no matter how small the meal might be. See yourself in that space. Take some deep breaths- exhale twice as long as you inhale- and sit with that thought.

Think back to a time when you felt good after a meal. See yourself content and satiated. It may have been a long time since you felt good about eating something. Your body and mind may have forgotten what that is like, and may feel uncomfortable at first. But that used to be your normal. Tell yourself that your body and mind need nourishment to be healthy.

You will learn to enjoy a good meal and the satiated feeling of a full stomach, but it will take practice and lots of positive self-talk. Start with small amounts of food and when that becomes comfortable (and it will, if you give it time) you can practice with larger meals.

My self-conversation goes something like this:

"You are going to be fine. One meal (or one bite) will not make you fat. You can do this, just relax. You are not fat."

I might have to say that over in my head a hundred times until I believe it. At first, I used such self-talk to get over the feeling of a full stomach until having a full stomach became my new norm. I still use this method on the occasional over-indulgence. Yes, sometimes I overeat, like most people without an eating disorder do. It is rare, but it happens- at a celebration meal, like Thanksgiving or Christmas dinner. And I still have to use self-talk to get past my fear of getting fat. The consequences of an overly full stomach remind me not to do it again. The pain reminds me I am only human. I tell myself it will pass in a few hours and I will be fine. And I am.

Purging removes the natural consequences of overeating. Allowing yourself to feel satiation and to be ok with it sets you up for success the next time you sit down for a meal. You may begin with one of five meals staying down, but say things to yourself like, "That's one more than last week. Good job!"

Are you willing to be uncomfortable until it becomes comfortable? That is what it will take to overcome your eating disorder. Start with small steps first, and build from there. Make up your mind to be uncomfortable for a little while. You decide what that looks like. Then sit with it for a while and ask yourself these questions.

What happened when I was uncomfortable?

_____

_____

_____

_____

How did I feel?

_____

_____

_____

_____

Could I do that again?

_____

Why or why not?

_____

_____

That is the process you will go through until the thing that makes you uncomfortable becomes your new normal. You didn't get into your eating disorder overnight, and you will not get out of it overnight. But you will get there, one baby step at a time. You may take two steps back and one step forward. Keep putting one foot in front of the other.

You can use self-talk whenever you feel anxious or stressed in any situation.

Here is one of my favorite exercises:

Remember when you were a kid. Did you ever wear a costume, pajamas, or a t-shirt that made you feel super-powered? Use that memory for this exercise.

Envision putting on a superhero cape or whatever empowers you.

What color is it?

What letter or words are there? Practice mentally putting on your super costume to help you believe you can do anything. Because, you can.

I tell myself in many situations: "I am a superhero or super ninja (i.e. supermom, super dad, super friend) and I can do this!"

You might want to do an art exercise for this chapter. You could find a superhero or ninja costume, cape, or T-shirt, pajamas and wear it sometimes.

Maybe you like to sew and could make your own cape or costume?

Draw or paint a picture of it?

Make a collage?

A sculpture?

Write a song?

A poem?

Involve whatever helps you to visualize your super powers and feels fun.

Imagine what you can do with these superpowers.

Imagine you are faster, stronger, or better than any human.

Imagine your superhero self is all-powerful.

Now tell yourself, "You are a superhero (super-ninja) and you can do anything."

You have power over your eating disorder or whatever you want to overcome. Now tell yourself you are that hero! You can do this.

Other things you can say to yourself:

This is only temporary and will soon pass. I can do this for five minutes (or one/two minutes).

I can do this.

I am strong enough to do this.

I am allowed to eat good things.

This meal won't make me fat.

I believe in me and I can do this.

I deserve good things and this is good for me.

This uncomfortable feeling will pass.

Keep going- this will soon become the norm.

When you accomplish the smallest feat, tell yourself how well you did!

Practice with non-food related situations as well. This exercise will increase your confidence and improve your feelings about yourself. The better you feel about you, the more confidence you gain in every area of your life.

Here are some things you can say to yourself:

You did good.

Well done.

Look at you go.

You can do this.

You are so strong.

You are so smart.

Good job.

Keep going, you can do this.

You go, girl (boy or whatever pronoun you choose)!

You got this.

This is your moment.

I'm so proud of you.

You are doing better every time.

Once you feel comfortable doing things you never thought possible, you can take it to the next level.

Lean into that uncomfortable feeling, even if it's only for a minute at a time. Spend a little time with the uncomfortable feeling. This is hard work, so be patient with yourself.

Remember, when you first meet new people or do something new, it feels a little uncomfortable until you get used to them or the situation. That comfortable space is where you want to go, but to get there, it will feel unnatural for a while.

Ask yourself:

What is the worst that can happen?

_____

_____

_____

What if I stay in this uncomfortable space for a little longer?

_____

_____

_____

Was that so bad?

_____

Could I do this just a bit longer next time?

_____

I used the superhero exercise recently to help me get ready for an evening out. My time management skills are lacking, so I have to plan ahead to be ready on time. But on this particular evening, I had about half of the time I needed to get ready. At first, I became anxious and stressed (which slowed me down more).

So, I talked to myself and said something like this:

"You are a superhero and you can do this! You are faster than any human on earth." I kept telling myself this as I got ready in record time. It was empowering and fun to imagine myself as a superhero, able to do things I normally couldn't. Yes, I got ready in record time, and instead of feeling anxious, I felt happy.

At first, self-talk may seem silly, but with time and practice, you will gain confidence, feel empowered, and be able to talk yourself through situations that would normally make you fall apart emotionally.

Self-talk is different from saying positive things or not criticizing yourself. It is talking to yourself like a patient friend, talking through uncomfortable feelings or situations and leading your mind where you want your body to go. Where your mind dwells, your body follows. You decide where you want to go and what thoughts you allow to lead you. Talking to yourself is the way to get to a better place where you are healthy, happy and free of your eating disorder.

RECOVERY LESSON #6:

You are not your body

> "Your body is not the real you. It's just the physical
> house you live in. The real you is your spirit, which
> will live on forever."
> **~David Berg**

Did you notice in this book that I use phrases to separate myself from my body or my brain?

Examples from the text: *My body is highly sensitive. My body reacted wildly. My body betrayed me. There was one way out, according to my brain. Numbers confused my brain.*

Do you know why?

Because I have learned to separate myself from my body. If I get sick, it's not *me* that is ill, it's my body. You, as in your spirit or personality, are not your body. You take up residence in your body, but it is not you. It's a physical vehicle you drive around.

If you believe you are mind, body, and spirit, then your mind, or your brain, is not you either. That is why I said that numbers confused my brain instead of numbers confused me.

You can like yourself, and not like your body- or parts of your body. For me, that idea helped me a lot in my recovery. Once I separated my body from me, it was easier to be objective.

Example: Muscle Fibers

My arms are short, with long muscle fibers.

Some people have long arms, with long muscle fibers. Some have long arms with short muscle fibers, or vice versa. How do you tell if you have long or short muscle fibers? Hold out an arm and look at your biceps area, from where the muscle meets the elbow to just below your shoulder. If the biceps muscle extends all the way, you have long muscle fibers. If the biceps muscle stops part of the way, you have short muscle fibers. It works the same way for muscles in your legs. Having either long or short muscle fibers isn't good or bad, it just is.

Long biceps muscle fibers can get much larger than small muscle fibers because they cover a larger area, but short biceps muscle fibers peak at the biceps much easier. Why does this matter? To you, it probably doesn't, unless you are into body-building. To me, it mattered a lot.

Back in the 1980s, when women's bodybuilding became popular, Cory Everson and Rachel McLish were the top contenders.
Rachel, my idol, had short muscle fibers in her arms and Cory
Everson had long muscled fibers. Rachel could never build
biceps as large as Cory could, but to me, her arms looked
much better. They were smaller, thinner, with a nice peak (like
the tip of a mountain) at the biceps. That is only my opinion.
I wanted to look like her, but I had arms like Cory. Bummer.

If bodybuilding contestants had been judged solely on basic
muscularity, Cory would have won every competition she
entered. Bodybuilders were scored based on a judge's pref-
erence, though, and Rachel often won competitions because
her body was feminine, lean, and more to their liking. To me,
she was a ten. She had long arms and legs, lean hips, and a
long narrow waist.

Nothing is ever going to change my genetic make-up. I am
stuck with short arms, and when I work them, they develop
big muscles and are hard to keep lean- and this reality bothers
me. In fact, ever since I reached puberty, I have hated how my
arms look, and how women's bodies hold on to fat, on the back
of their arms and under them. The only times that how my
arms looked didn't bother me were the times I weighed under
a hundred pounds, because at that weight, most of my body
fat was gone.

How I feel about my arms has been- and is- my secret truth,
but it doesn't have to define me, depress me, or cast me into

darkness. I may not like my arms, but I still like myself. My arms are not me; they are a part of my body. And I choose to accept them.

When you tell one of your painful secrets to yourself or to someone you trust, it loses its power over you. Getting it out in the open allows for healing to enter into that area of your life. As long as you hide a secret away, it also holds onto you, which is why I encourage you to seek professional help. They can help you to uncover the hard secrets in your own life and provide a safe place for you to talk about things. Keeping a secret can be a burden, especially when it's your own.

Recently, I felt I needed extra support while dealing with a family issue, and I sought out a therapist for the first time in many years- and I'm so glad I did! This woman has helped me to discover and release feelings I've had trapped inside. I forgot how good it can feel to work with a professional. If you need someone to tell you to seek help, this is me telling you to reach out.

At different times in our lives, we may find we need additional help. There is no shame in having or needing a counselor, no matter how old you are. The important thing is to allow yourself to feel things, and to express them and find healthy ways to do that. Virtual therapy appointments are now widely available and can expand the list of professionals you can choose from to help you. Find someone you connect with and trust. Even if it has been years since you felt the need, life changes and circumstances shift and you may feel the need for support at various times.

After years of practice, I recently took acceptance of my arms a step further and turned that acceptance into gratitude. I was watching a couple dance, and I noticed how petite the woman was. Her arms were long and lean. At first, I wished my arms looked like hers, but upon further inspection, I noticed how thin she was. In fact, her body looked like that of an adolescent. Her arms weren't just thin, they looked frail. She was smiling on the outside, but that disposition didn't look genuine. It seemed like she had painted on that smile, and I wondered if she had an eating disorder because she looked like she weighed about ninety pounds.

The more I observed her, the more grateful I became for my muscular arms that had shape and contour. To be a healthy woman felt good.

I even said to my arms, "I like that you are not frail. I feel grateful for my powerful arms."

The second part of the lesson in this example was that I realized a fault in my thinking. At first, I was thinking that a childlike, undernourished body was better than a strong woman's body. And in that moment, seeing health for what it is, I gave myself permission to be a mature woman who liked her arms.

Then I told myself, "Good job! That was awesome mental work you just did. I'm proud of you!"

Are there parts of your body you don't like? Why?

Pay attention to how you speak to yourself or to others about that part of your body, because you are listening. Your body is not you; it is where you take up residence.

"And I said to my body softly, 'I want to be your friend.' It took a long breath and replied, 'I have been waiting my whole life for this." — Nayyirah Waheed.

RECOVERY LESSON #7:

Stop criticizing yourself

> "You have been criticizing yourself for years and it hasn't worked. Try approving of yourself and see what happens."
> ~*Louise Hay.*

In a passage I recall from a book by one of my bodybuilder idols, Rachel McLish, she was speaking of body types, and she wrote that she had an ugly, pear-shaped body. Her self-analysis was her perception, but not reality. I thought she had a perfect body. The very things I thought were her best features, she thought were her worst.

The way you see your body is your perception. I may not like my arms, but it is only in my perception that, to me, they look good or bad. Separating who you are from how you look or think you look is a tremendous step forward in your recovery.

With bodybuilding, I could change the way my body looked. I couldn't change my short muscles, but I could replace body fat with muscle, sculpting it like an artist. Exercise helped me deal with parts of my body that I didn't like. It took years spent hour-by-hour in the gym, eating right, and dedication to achieve the results I wanted. For me, bodybuilding was a very positive part of my life most of the time. Instead of starving myself, I transformed my body with weight lifting.

There was a point when bodybuilding became a substitute for my eating disorder, though. The same obsession that drove my eating disorder found another outlet in exercise. Before I had my other two children and got married, I was impassioned with working out and wanted to compete in my first body-building competition. The same messed-up thinking patterns I'd developed toward eating applied to my workout routine. My hyperfocus on what I ate, my workout routines, and my progress building muscle resulted in a lack of balance in my life.

Do you find yourself in a similar situation, hyperfocused on your body and how it looks?

What could you focus on instead?

Shifting focus to activities that aren't related to your body can help you find balance. A creative hobby instead of a physical activity might be just what you need. Spend some time thinking about it.

Why not take an art class instead of dance?

Maybe you always wanted to play the violin or guitar?

Learn to paint?

Take a writing class?

Acting lessons?

The choices are endless, so dig deep and start looking around. Think outside the box…

Learn a new language?

Write in script?

Plant a garden?

Decorate a space?

Luckily for me, at that time, I had my daughter to consider and care for, and that responsibility stopped me from competing, and I remember the moment I made a conscious decision not to go down that road. My daughter and I were sitting at the table one evening and I fixed her a piece of toast with butter, cinnamon, and sugar to go with her cup of hot cocoa. This was a rare treat, and she giggled with delight.

"Here, mom," she said, holding a piece of sticky toast to my mouth, smiling. My first reaction was to refuse it, but the look on her face when I turned away touched my heart. It took me about two seconds to change my mind.

To compete would have meant there would be no more of such treats for me. In order to reach peak condition, I had to monitor my carbohydrate and fat intake strictly. I realized how self-centered that pursuit would be. Everything in my life would center on diet, workouts, and me, me, me- so I poured myself a cup of hot cocoa, took a bite of her toast, then made us another piece. It was better, I thought, to enjoy these sorts of moments than to compete in any bodybuilding competition. That was an excellent decision.

No matter how much I'd changed my body composition with weight lifting, I still criticized myself. There was always something I could find fault in. My legs were too thick, I was too short, my calves were too small... The judgment never ended.

Societies (and different cultures) create their own ideas of what is physically attractive in a person. We might find it abhorrent to put large round discs in our lower lips, disfiguring our face, but that might be what another culture sees as beautiful. The ideal of beauty changes around the world. In our society, it can change from month-to-month. What was in style last year or last month is now out of style. Pressure to conform and a corresponding belief that we are less than what our idea of perfection is leads to self-criticizing (shaming).

Yet, we are each different: no two of us are the same. What a boring world it would be if we were each molded into either a Barbie or a Ken doll. It might be fun for a short while, but ultimately, we'd be boring.

A gigantic step in my recovery was to stop criticizing myself. Like stopping my negative self-talk, catching myself in the act of self-criticism and replacing it with positive comments took practice. The first thing I taught myself was how to accept a compliment. This is harder than you might think. Have you mastered this skill? Give it a go.

The next time someone says anything complimentary to you, note your reaction. To respond with anything other than a genuine smile, and a "thank you" means you have work to do.

Usually, it goes something like this:

"I like your dress!"

"Oh, this is old thing? I just dug it out of the bottom of my closet."

For me, it's usually related to my hair:

"I love your hair!"

"Thanks, but it's a lot of work."

Ever hear someone receive a compliment well? I have. It blows my mind. They don't downgrade the compliment. They don't add or subtract anything to it- they just appreciate the compliment and smile or say thank you.

So, I practiced taking a compliment until I could react positively. My goal was to accept a compliment without replying with a derogatory comment. At first, I would react as I always did, with some downgrade to myself. But when I caught myself doing that, I'd have a talk with myself.

"Next time, just say thank you. The way so-and-so does."

And pretty soon, I could accept a compliment without a downgrade.

Sometimes I slip and find myself back in old habits, but then I remind myself to just accept the compliment the next time. The old me would beat me up verbally over any slip-up. Instead of striving for perfection, my new goal is to make progress in a positive direction.

You can do the same thing with self-criticism. Recognize first that you do it, and then write in your journal what you tell yourself. Don't spend too much time writing negative things down; just jot a few comments so that you become aware of how often you are criticizing yourself. Soon, you will catch yourself mentally and can turn your criticisms into positivisms.

Write some positivisms for yourself. Make a list, even if you can only come up with one item for it to start. Need ideas? I bet your friends, acquaintances, or co-workers give you positivisms. Add those comments to your list if you don't yet have any of your own. Focus on anything positive about yourself.

Maybe you have pretty hands or beautiful fingernails, or good-looking feet, or nice eyes… Find one thing about your appearance that you like, even if it's your eyelashes. No matter how insignificant it seems, find some physical attribute about yourself that you like.

For me, one such body part I now appreciate is my neck. It's long and slender. I used to think it was ugly. I called it my "turtle neck", until someone commented on my lovely neck. They wished they had it. Really? Now I wear clothes and a hairstyle to show it off. What I once thought was ugly, someone else saw as beautiful.

I give compliments to myself and to others. If I think someone has beautiful hair, a great shirt, or an attractive purse, I tell them, because maybe they need to hear it. A few words might just make their day or their year. Have you ever held onto a compliment and rehearsed it over and over in your mind?

I once heard an oft-criticized husband say to a friend when he thought no one was listening, "That lady told me she liked my eyes. That compliment was enough to keep me going for a year!" His wife had fallen into a habit of criticizing him, and it only took one compliment to make his year. Imagine what positivisms can do for not only you, but for others.

RECOVERY LESSON #8:

Taking responsibility

> "When you think everything is someone else's fault, you will suffer a lot. When you realize that everything springs only from yourself, you will learn both peace and joy."
> **~Dalai Lama.**

This is a big lesson. Are you ready for this one?

I spent a lot of my life suffering, blaming others, and feeling sorry for myself until one day a friend said some harsh words to me.

"Stop feeling sorry for yourself. So, your childhood sucked- so what? There are many other people that have suffered worse."

Those words pissed me off for a long time- until I realized he was right. I'd been feeling sorry for myself, hanging onto my "story" for years. Poor me.

When you focus on your own suffering, you cannot see the suffering in others, which may be much worse than anything you could imagine. I've heard many stories similar to my own, and I realize how fortunate I was.

One of my mentor friends taught me two simple questions to use in any situation where I feel wronged.

"What was my part in it?"

"What could I have done differently?"

I'm not talking about situations in childhood, or of domestic violence, where one person dominates another physically or emotionally so that they have no choice or power in a situation. But these questions apply to situations involving adults in mutual relationships, whether they work, live, or exist together.

As long as I blamed my mom, my brothers, or my dad for my problems, my eating disorder held me captive. Bad things happen to good people, and good things happen to bad people. That's life. However, we have the power to decide what to do with the cards that are dealt to us.

Example: I couldn't make my dad love me the way I needed to be loved, but I could love and respect him, regardless. My actions toward him were my choice.

Such behavior is the exact opposite of what your pride will tell you to do, or what society might say. They want you to play the victim. We all do it- some more than others- but everyone has done it. People who take responsibility for their lives recognize unfortunate or bad situations and choose to control their reactions to them, while victims don't. First, you must learn to recognize when you are playing the victim or blaming others.

To take responsibility for your own actions, regardless of what others say or do, is a skill that few will master. I haven't mastered it, but I'm getting better at it.

Here's the thing. The only control you have in this world is over yourself and how you react. You don't control the weather, peace, war, or what happens moment to moment. And most of all, you can't control anyone else. People will do what they do, say what they say, go where they want. They will lie, steal and cheat or live, laugh and love. But you can choose what you do and how you respond to things.

Example: Just because I apologize to someone doesn't mean they will forgive me. I can't control what they do, only what I do which feels right, by apologizing.

How someone responds to you is not your business, because you can't control them. But how you respond to others, that is your business. When people don't respond the way we want them to or think they should, we get upset.

Think you have control over your reactions to others?

I play a little game with myself from time to time to see how well I've learned this lesson. My goal in this exercise is to pass more often than I fail.

One of my favorite activities is hiking. When I'm out on the trails, I make it a point to yield to traffic. Even if I have the right of way, I try to get out of the way when I can- especially for mountain bikers, because I used to ride, and I know how annoying it is to stop or slow down for pedestrians. The lesson part comes from my expectations of their reaction. How do I react when they don't say thank you? More times than not, I grumble if they don't react the way I want them to, and I smile when they do. This exercise tells me a lot about myself and where I am on my journey.

Try it yourself, in the car, on the street, in the store, or with your friends and family. Do something nice for someone with no expectation of a response or reaction. You could wave and smile at passersby. Let a driver go in front of you, or pull a grocery cart out or put one away for a stranger. Open a door for someone, let them ahead of you in line, or give them a compliment. Offer an elderly neighbor a ride to a doctor's appointment, mow their lawn or sweep their sidewalk. Brush the snow off a co-worker or neighbor's car, pet sit, or buy someone flowers for no reason at all.

How does it make you feel if they don't react the way you want them to?

_____

_____

The way you respond to their reaction is your business and you're responsible for it. And it's the only thing you control in this world. Maybe you could make up your own game to gauge your reaction to things you can't control. Remember, the goal is not perfection, just self-actualization. When you realize you can't control other people or what they do, you will be on a healing path.

I remind myself of this concept often. When I think I've learned the lesson, I play my game, only to find there is more work for me to do on myself. We are all works in progress, and we never arrive. Life is in the living, not the arriving. Give yourself some grace in the process of healing and keep going. You are doing so well!

Now that you understand you are responsible for your actions and reactions and can't control others, it is time to take personal responsibility a little further.

Have you ever thought about how your eating disorder affects those around you?

_____

_____

Why or why not?

_____

_____

_____

Have you asked your friends/family/spouse or partner how it affects them?

_____

Chances are that your eating disorder affects those around you, whether or not you want it to.

Here are some questions to ask yourself:

How does my eating disorder affect those around me?

_____

_____

_____

_____

_____

How do I feel about that?

_____

_____

_____

_____

Are there things I could do to help my friends/family/spouse/partner deal with my eating disorder?

_____

_____

_____

_____

_____

Do I use my eating disorder to gain attention?

_____

Do I use my eating disorder to feel in control?

_____

Why?

_____

_____

_____

_____

_____

Is there someone in my life that doesn't give me the attention I want/deserve or crave?

_____

_____

Have I ever discussed this unmet need with that person?

_____

Why or why not?

_____

_____

_____

What would that conversation sound like?

_____

_____

_____

What would that conversation look like?

_____

_____

_____

Do I feel safe enough in my relationship/s to discuss my unmet needs?

_____

What would make me feel safe enough to discuss my unmet needs with another?

_____

_____

_____

Are there other ways to get the attention I want/deserve/need from others besides using my eating disorder?

_____

What would those other ways look like?

_____

_____

_____

_____

Maybe others have caused you pain (emotional and/or physical), exerted control over you, or made decisions that affected you negatively (through a divorce, an unwanted move, or negative comments). I get that. That part is their responsibility. But this chapter is about you and your responsibility.

Do you blame others for your eating disorder?

_____

Do you use others as an excuse to continue in your disorder?

_____

How?

_____

_____

_____

_____

Once you become an adult, you are responsible for your actions. **If you are an adolescent or younger, please reach out to a trusted person in authority that can help you find professional help. Especially if you do not feel safe at home or in a relationship.**

If you are a friend/spouse/sibling/parent of a person with an eating disorder, here are some questions for you:

Have my behaviors/words/actions contributed to this person's eating disorder?

_____

How do I know?

_____

_____

_____

_____

Did my behaviors/words/actions make a positive impact on this person?

_____

Have I ever asked them if my behaviors/words/actions hurt them?

_____

Did I ever inquire about what they might need/want from me?

_____

Why or why not?

_____

_____

_____

_____

Has it ever crossed my mind that I could have contributed to their eating disorder?

_____

Why or why not?

_____

_____

_____

Have I ever asked the person with the eating disorder if they feel that my behavior/words/actions contributed to their disorder?

_____

At first, the questions related to this step may be too big for you or anyone around you to dig into. You and/or they may need the help of a counselor to guide you through this conversation. That's ok. I told you this was a **BIG** lesson. It may take months or years for you to fully recognize when you are no longer playing the victim and are taking responsibility for your actions. It's alright to take small steps through this lesson, each as you feel ready.

Look at how far you have come already! Focus on each step you take forward and celebrate.

RECOVERY LESSON #9:

Stop taking things personally

> "Personal importance, or taking things personally, is
> the maximum expression of selfishness because we
> make the assumption that everything is about me."
> ~*Miguel Ruiz*

We don't need anyone to teach us how to be selfish because it
is part of our human nature. How often have you heard someone say, "If that was me, I'd do this or that." Do you know why
people say that? Because they relate everything to themselves.
Even when it's not about them. Guilty!

If you want to be miserable in life, assume everything is about
you. Many people go through life doing that. Especially those
with eating disorders. I know I used my eating disorder to cope
with life and to escape my emotional pain. But it took much

longer for me to discover how selfish it was. I became hyper-focused on myself- how I looked, what I ate, and how much I weighed. Everything was about me, which led me into the habit of taking things personally.

Examine your own behaviors and thought patterns to decide where you live on the selfish scale. It is hard to admit that we are being selfish. But that was one of my truths and until I owned it, I couldn't get past my destructive behavior.

You may not consider your behavior selfish. It may or may not be. That is not my place to tell you. If you want to get free of your eating disorder, asking yourself some tough questions will be part of your recovery. You get to decide when you are ready for each lesson.

And asking yourself if you are being selfish is one of those hard questions. But I encourage you to ask yourself the hard questions when you feel ready. If you find yourself taking things personally, it's a sign that deep down, you think everything is about you.

Here is an example of taking things personally: Let's say someone doesn't call or answer right away when we reach out. We may assume they are ignoring us and get upset (that's making their response or lack of response about us before we know the facts).

Or: Two people are talking and looking our way. We may assume they are talking negatively about us. We may get upset, which could lead to us to internalize our feelings and lead to a binge, a purge, or starvation- first, as a punishment for ourselves (they don't love me, they don't like me, I'm not good enough etc.), or as a punishment towards them (you don't love me, you don't like me, or you don't give me the attention I need).

What does it feel like when I take things personally?

_____

_____

_____

_____

What if I assumed things were not about me until I know the facts? What would that look like?

_____

_____

_____

_____

What would that feel like?

_____

_____

_____

_____

Another example: Some challenging things occur at work/ home/in your personal life and you feel the need to speak to someone. You start by reaching out with an email. There is no response for several hours, so you send them a message. There is still no response, so you call them after several hours and leave a voicemail. Still, you receive no response. You have two choices. Assume this is about you (take it personally) or assume it's not about you and is circumstantial (maybe they aren't in today, maybe they didn't see the message, etc.)

If you assume it is about me (i.e. they are ignoring me, they don't care about me, they don't like me), you may get angry, hurt or resentful and cause yourself undue stress, anxiety, or worry, which can trigger your eating disorder.

Not taking the lack of response personally (it isn't about me) looks much different. In this scenario, you reason that something must have happened that caused your manager/friend/family/spouse/significant other not to reply. Maybe they were busy and saw the message but didn't have time to reply. Or maybe they were sick today. Or maybe they never even saw your message?

When you don't take things personally, it allows time and space for you to learn the facts about unexpected actions and respond accordingly.

Here are a series of questions I ask myself to help make sure I'm not taking things personally- not just at work, but in life, and with relationships.

What is the story I'm telling myself about this situation?

_____

_____

_____

_____

_____

Is it the truth?

_____

How do I know it's the truth?

_____

_____

_____

Then you can use reason and tell yourself, "There might be good reasons for the silence (or situation) that I know nothing about."

Slowing down to ask yourself these questions takes time and practice, but is worthwhile.

This lesson is intended to help you learn to not take things so personally, and also to help you discern what thought patterns you may practice that keep you stuck in your disorder.

Instead of assuming a non-response is personal, you can ask the other person.

"Hey, did you see my message?"

"Hey, you didn't respond to my message. Did you see it yet?"

Of course, there are times others make things personal and attack us, and that is a different scenario.

I suggest you find and work with a qualified professional to learn the difference between the two. A good counselor will help you to recognize when someone else's communication to you is threatening and help you to develop healthy ways to react in those situations, as well as help you to see and stop taking things personal when they aren't.

The **What If** game can help you to not take everything so personally. It's a mental game I play to realign my thinking. When I get caught up in assuming situations are about me, I challenge myself to turn my perspective around.

Let's say someone doesn't reply right away to your message, and your first thought is, "They don't like me, so they aren't answering."

Or you think, "I did something that caused them to ignore me. It's all my fault."

Or "They are ignoring me. They must hate me."

Instead, you say to yourself:

What if they simply didn't see my message?

What if their phone went dead?

A healthy response might be: *I'm sure there is a good reason for their lack of response. I will reach out again and make sure that they are alright.*

Can you think of other responses that might help you to not take things so personally?

_____

_____

_____

_____

How do you feel when you say those responses to yourself instead of taking things personally?

_____

_____

_____

_____

You can even say something funny like:

What if a giant caterpillar ate their phone/computer?

What if an elephant sat on their phone and it's broke?

What if the Easter Bunny took their phone/computer so they can't answer?

When we take things personally, we assume another's response (or lack of response) is about us, and often related to something I did or didn't do. We might think they are punishing us, ignoring us, or purposely hurting us, because it's all about me, right?

The reality may differ from your perception, though, and the other person probably isn't aware of the pain or struggle you are going through because you took their actions personally.

In truth, there might be a simple explanation for an unexpected response. When we take things personally, we assume someone's action or non-action is all about us.

Most of the time, they probably were busy, didn't see the message or the call, or they even forgot to reply because they got distracted by the eight million other things that happened since they received your message.

When in doubt, ask.

"Did you see my last message?" or "Did you get my call?" and, "Is everything ok? I didn't hear from you, and I was concerned."

Assume it's not about you until you know the facts.

The road to recovery has steep hills, deep valleys, and hard speed bumps, so take it slow and give yourself the time and space you need to deal with each lesson. This particular lesson may be hard to face, but you can do it!

As a parent, I've played out the most horrific scenarios in my mind when one of my children came home a few minutes late, or I couldn't get in contact with them. Have you ever done that? I'm so good at it, I have made myself cry sometimes, certain I would never see them again. We live in a harsh world and the worst can happen, but needless stress and worry come with our negative thoughts. What we think about something can cause us trauma long before or after it happens.

RECOVERY LESSON #10:

Live in harmony

)|●|(

> "Happiness is when what you think, what you say, and
> what you do are in harmony."
> ~*Muhatma Ghandi*

Everyone talks about finding balance in life. A truly balanced life, by definition, would have you allocating time and energy equally in all areas of your life. Harmony, however, is what I believe most of us are seeking. I looked up its definition in the Merriam-Webster dictionary.

Harmony: Pleasing arrangement of parts.

Wouldn't it be nice to have a life that had a pleasing arrangement of every part?

What would that look like for you?

_____

_____

_____

_____

For me, living in harmony leads to happiness. How can living in harmony lead to happiness? I'm glad you asked.

The chapter's lead quote reminds me to examine my thoughts, actions, and motivations. If I believe one thing but act or think in opposition to that belief, I will experience inner struggle, perhaps without even knowing it.

An easy way to describe disharmony is like so: if your thoughts, feelings, words, and actions are not aligned, you will feel unbalanced. If you are unbalanced (off center), you will feel uncomfortable.

Lack of harmony in one area of your life will show up in other areas of your life, which ultimately will cause you to feel unhappy. And you might not even know why you feel unhappy, just that you do. The more you are out of harmony, the more unhappy you will feel.

Asking yourself the question "Am I in harmony?" will lead you to examine your life on a deeper level. This is a practice that you can learn. The more you do it, the better you will get at recognizing when harmony within yourself exists and when it doesn't.

I ask myself often if my actions, thoughts, and speech are in alignment. If the answer is no, I reexamine where I need to change something. Remember, learning to find harmony is a practice. It is becoming aware of areas in your life where you need more work, and allowing yourself the grace to practice realigning your words, thoughts, and actions.

Since we can't live a perfectly balanced life, I prefer to think of being in harmony as staying centered, like placing yourself in the middle of a circle. All things that are part of your life surround you like pieces of a pie: work, sleep, eating, meal prep, cooking, cleaning, entertainment, relaxation, play, fun, creative endeavors, sex and exercise.

In each of our lives, there are parts of it we have to do, parts we don't like to do, parts we do like to do, parts we do for others, parts we do because we feel we have to, and parts we want to do more.

If we spend too much of our time on things we have to do and don't enjoy, we may lose our sense of being centered- which can lead us into unhappiness, or even worse, depression, resentment, anger, hostility, or loneliness, which keep us out of harmony.

In order to be in harmony, the slices of your life pie need to include enough of the things you like to do and want to do, but not too many. Living for too much fun can lead to laziness, financial ruin, and the loss of relationships, work, or self-respect, while living for too much work, or things we have to do, without allowing some fun, exercise, and creativity in your life can lead to resentment and burn-out.

As you age, have a family, take a new job, or move across town or the world, your pie will look different, depending on what stage of life you are in. Raising a family and caring for elders or others can take an inordinate amount of our pie. This lesson is about learning to stay in harmony, no matter what stage of life you are in.

You will know you are not in harmony when there are too many pieces of one kind filling the pie of your life and not enough from other types.

Let's say you have the goal of becoming financially independent and retiring at 60, but you don't have a plan. You don't save regularly, and you don't know how much money you will need to retire comfortably. You fail to study investments or educate yourself, preventing you from achieving your goal. The mismatch between your financial desires and your actions creates a lack of harmony within you. Although you express a desire for financial independence, your lack of effort in the area shows otherwise. Get it?

Maybe you hate your job. You dream of better pay, more fulfillment in your work, and a more positive work environment, but you don't apply for any new positions or study the job market to see what is available in your area. You aren't thinking about what kind of work you might be interested in and you aren't looking into furthering your education. Instead, all you do is complain and settle for less than you are sure you are worth. You are out of harmony.

Now, let's relate this lesson to your eating disorder.

Being out of harmony in any area of your life can lead to an eating disorder, or magnify an existing disorder. And eating disorders, regardless of the type, demonstrate a lack of harmony in their practitioner's life.

Here are some common traits that characterize each fundamental type of eating disorder.

Anorexics: People in this group are super strict and hard on themselves, not only by limiting their food intake, but by adhering to an ever-increasing exercise routine. They often live by a stringent set of self-imposed rules, have little fun, do not allow themselves to enjoy life, and feel like no matter what they do, they are never good enough.

Bulimics (binge/purge): People in this group stuff their feelings inside, leave emotions undealt with, avoid confrontation, isolate themselves, and blame others for their problems.

Bingers: People in this group use food as an escape, handle stress poorly, have low self-esteem, and exhibit little or no self-control once a binge starts.

You might have a combination of all the of traits and types listed above, as I did. Because I lived in that way for thirteen years, I get to say: *I was so out of harmony*!

Can you see the lack of harmony in each lifestyle? It is easy to see a lack of harmony in others, but what about in ourselves?

Let's start with your own pie and see what that looks like. In this exercise, I want you to make a list of all of the main activities that fill your life. Next, let's create a pie divided into as many pieces as it takes to reflect the activities that fill your life, with you in the center. Size the pieces according to how much time you spend doing each activity. You might add a piece or two for things that you want to do but that you don't spend any time doing now.

You can use any medium you want to illustrate this pie. Paint, pencil, pen, watercolor, pastel, construction paper or whatever you like. You could create a 3-D pie with various materials.

Look at the division of parts.

How much time do you spend working?

_____

Preparing meals?

_____

Watching TV?

_____

Playing video games?

_____

Exercising?

_____

Eating?

_____

Sex (if age appropriate)?

_____

Reading?

_____

At church?

_____

Sleeping?

_____

Being creative?

_____

Having fun?

_____

Spending time with family/friends/spouse/partner?

_____

How much time do you spend on activities related to your eating disorder (i.e. bingeing, purging, prepping meals, grocery shopping, exercising)?

_____

Do you see any huge disparities in your pie?

_____

What are they?

_____

Does your pie include pleasing activities that are fun, creative, and connect you with others?

_____

Why/Why not?

_____

_____

_____

Now, think about what a harmonious pie would look like and create that pie (a pleasing arrangement of parts).

What differences are there between the pies?

_____

_____

_____

What would it feel like if your life were more harmonious?

_____

_____

_____

What could you do to achieve a more harmonious life?

_____

_____

_____

The first step towards balancing your life is being aware of where you are, and where you want to be. Until you recognize when and where a lack of harmony exists in your life, you won't be able to change anything. Start with just one piece of your pie that is out of harmony, and work on balancing that area. As you gain more harmony in your life, it will help you to see other areas within that might be out of harmony, and will make it easier for you to recognize and remedy these imbalances. Take small steps at first, and then you can take bigger steps as you progress. Any step towards increased harmony in your life is a success, so celebrate each improvement, no matter how small it seems.

RECOVERY LESSON #11:

Uncovering emotional layers

> "Healing is like an onion. As you process through one layer of trauma to release the pain and heal, a new layer will surface. One layer after another layer will bring up new issues to focus on. Pace yourself. Only focus on one layer at a time."
> **~Dan Arcuri**

Earlier, I used an onion to describe the layers of an eating disorder. Think about an onion. On the outside, all you see is a round bulb with a stem on top. If you hold it in your hand, you feel the first layers, thin, paper-like, on the outside. You might be able to easily rub off parts of those first layers with the tips of your fingers, depending on how long the onion has been out of the ground. Other layers will be tougher to get through.

Picture yourself as an onion.

You have layers that wrap around you, containing all of your life inside of you. To get to the inside layers, you must remove the outside layers first. That is what recovery is: peeling back one layer of your life at a time and dealing with all of the emotional stuff in that layer until you discover the next layer.

You will peel back a layer and think you're done, only to find it attached to another. The first few layers are the easiest to remove, but the deeper you go, the thicker the layers are. You can't get to the center layers unless you cut into the onion, or peel the layers one by one. Cutting is painful, so let's be gentle and start by peeling away layer by layer.

To heal, you must peel away your own layers. You need to find the first emotional layer to get started. You might not understand what that is, or how to start, and that's why working with a professional therapist is important. They can help you uncover the emotional layers in your life one by one and heal them until you are ready to work on the next layer.

Your journey might start with scratching that first outside layer. That might be enough to work on for some time. That's ok. Don't worry about getting to the other layers. Focus on dealing with the first layer, or part of that layer.

Here are some ideas that might help you get started finding the layers of your onion.

Visualize yourself (or the eating disorder, if that's easier) as an onion with emotional layers.

What does it look like? (Plump, elongated, round, top-heavy, long-stemmed, short-stemmed, no stem)

_____

What color is it?

_____

How many layers do you think are inside?

_____

Are you ready to peel back a layer or just a small part of one?

_____

Why?

_____

_____

_____

What would help you be ready to peel the layers?

_____

_____

_____

What do you think is inside the first layer?

_____

_____

_____

Do you know what the other layers are?

You could do a creative exercise to help you visualize the onion. Think you are not creative? Start with a real onion if you need to, or a picture of an onion.

When you let your creative mind work, it can help heal you from the inside out. As you focus on a project or creation, it can tap into feelings you are unaware of. Creativity gets you in touch with your inner child, the part of yourself that is unhindered and likes to have fun. That is the part you want to rekindle.

The goal of this exercise is to create an onion to represent the emotional layers in you. As you uncover each layer, you can add them to your design. You can have more than one onion—there are no rules here. Your onion doesn't need to be perfect or pretty. Let your onion be what it wants to be, whatever that is.

Here are some suggestions:

Draw an onion and label each layer as you peel it back, or what you think each layer might be. Use any medium you feel would represent your onion: paint, colored pencils, construction paper, decorations, jewelry, stencils, markers, wood, sticks, rocks. You get to choose. Let your creativity lead you in this exercise.

Maybe you start with a black onion, because that's how you feel inside. Or an onion that's turned brown on the inside.

You could create two onions, one for what you thought your emotional layers were, and one for what you discover the layers are.

Your onion could be textured with jewels, sparkles, dirt, or anything that you feel represents your layers. A papier mâché onion might be fun!

If you are a friend, family member, or partner of a person with an eating disorder, you can also make your own onion. In fact, I recommend that you do. You could make your own onion or create an onion together with that person. Let your imagination take over.

Maybe you could share your emotional layers with someone.

Who would you choose to share a layer with?

_____

What would that look like?

_____

_____

_____

Sound like?

_____

_____

_____

Feel like?

You could write a poem, a song about the onion layers and what they represent. The only rule is to make a representation of an onion to help you visualize your own emotional layers.

The longer you have had an eating disorder, the more layers you will have. Uncovering them is difficult and may be painful to face, unbearable perhaps, or so it will seem. The road to freedom and happiness is a process well worth the journey, but not without the price of admission. There is work and pain in progress.

Be gentle with yourself and with others. This is a lesson you can come back to months or even years later if new emotional layers reveal themselves. Do not rush, push, or pull yourself through an additional layer. Peel a layer as slowly as necessary. Each strip you peel back and deal with is progress, no matter how slow you go. This is hard work, so applaud yourself for each step you take!

RECOVERY LESSON #12:

Happiness is a choice

> "Whoever is happy will make others happy."
> ~*Anne Frank, The Diary of a Young Girl*

Ever meet someone who exudes happiness? No matter what happens to them, they find the good in others and their circumstances. I don't think we are born that way. I think that is a learned behavior. However, I think some people are more optimistic than others.

When I lived in Flagstaff, Arizona, there was a Walgreens store I dubbed the happiest place on earth. Two pharmacists that worked there were the friendliest girls I'd ever met. They smiled, greeted the customers happily, laughed, and I never heard them say a harsh word. Even when people were grouchy. Their happiness was infectious. When I went into that store, I started smiling, just watching them. They had joy, not that fake niceness that some people exude.

One day, I arrived at the counter to find them both in leg casts. One was on crutches, the other on one of those scooters used to get around on one leg. I'm sure they were both in pain. Limited in movement, stumbling into each other as they worked to fill my order, they were both laughing. While they were gleefully filling my prescription, I asked what happened. They both had had accidents, on different days, in different ways, with the same outcome: casts for six weeks. Me, I'd be miserable, whining away because of the pain and inconvenience, and because I couldn't exercise or get around easily. But those two?

They were like the Whos down in Dr. Suess's Whoville when the Grinch stole Christmas. Their happiness came not from outside of themselves or their circumstances, but from within. By that time in my life, I considered myself to be pretty happy. But they inspired me. I've thought of those girls for years and often tell that story because it had a profound impact on me. They made a choice to be happy despite challenging circumstances. And their joy spread to everyone that entered that store.

They did not choose to be hurt or in casts. Misfortune happened to them, regardless of whether they wanted it to or not. Life is like that. Shit happens. How we respond to what happens to us is the difference between being happy or being miserable. It's a choice. And when you choose to be happy, despite your circumstances, you will make others happy.

My eating disorders developed and continued because I wasn't happy inside. Turmoil, chaos, and depression are the weights I dragged around. I found myself trapped beneath layers of unfaced emotions which drove me to make decisions that created more unhappiness in my life. In order to be happy, I first had to deal with all the things that created my unhappiness. The more unhappy I was, the more disorder ruled my life. I was out of balance, lacked harmony, and felt unhappy most of the time. Now, I can say, I feel happy most days. Deliriously happy. But I spent years uncovering the layers of my unhappiness and doing the emotional work to arrive at where I am today.

Everyone wants to be happy, but most of us don't know how to achieve happiness or sustain it. The secret, for me, was peeling back one emotional layer at a time and dealing with each part as it revealed itself (see Lesson #11). Happiness is a choice we can make, but if you find yourself unable to feel happy, revisit Lesson #11 on uncovering emotional layers. You may have deep layers of pain you have not yet uncovered or healed from yet.

Questions you can ask:

Do I feel happy?

_____

Was there a time when I felt happy?

_____

Why/why not?

_____

_____

Do I want to be happy?

_____

Why/why not?

_____

_____

_____

Do I believe feeling happy is possible?

_____

What brings happiness to my life?

_____

Do I believe happiness is a choice?

_____

Why/why not?

_____

_____

_____

Could I choose to feel happy today?

_____

Is there anything I can find to be happy about right now?

_____

Do I know anyone that seems happy?

_____

Are they happy most of the time?

_____

Have I ever asked why they are happy?

_____

Could I ask them what it feels like to be happy?

_____

Do cheerful people make me feel happy?

_____

Why/why not?

_____

What could I do to make someone feel happy?

_____

_____

What could someone else do that might help me feel happy?

_____

_____

_____

_____

RECOVERY LESSON #13:

Speak your truth

> "There is a price to pay for speaking the truth. There
> is a bigger price for living a lie."
> ~ *Cornel West.*

The first time I spoke my truth after a meal, I realized the power of it. If hiding from my true feelings kept me in bondage to my eating disorder, maybe putting them out there would help free me.

"Can I go throw up now?" I asked candidly. It was a joke, but a gigantic step toward my recovery. I wanted to go throw up after a meal with friends. They knew of my disorder, so it wasn't a surprise that I might do that. Instead of hiding my truth from anyone, I spoke it out loud. Everyone stared at me, not knowing how to react until I laughed.

"Just kidding. I won't, but I want to," I said. "Thought you all should know."

Light exposes darkness. Saying what I felt instead of covering up my desire to purge took the power away from the desire. Of course, not everyone can handle hearing such truth, so you must know your audience before blurting out such things. For me, it was being gut level honest with myself and my friends. It felt so freeing! I still do that sometimes, when I've eaten too much, and feel uncomfortable.

The difference now is that I know the feeling of being full will pass if I let it. I still want to purge after a big meal, but if I hide those feelings from myself or others, I stay in the lie. If I speak my truth, I'm not hiding that impulse. It's out there.

Sometimes I say things to myself like, "I'm so full. It makes me want to go throw up."

Once I've admitted it to myself or others, then I talk myself out of it. Think about what you would say to a friend that shared such a secret.

What would you say to them?

_____

_____

_____

_____

Example: "You are feeling uncomfortable now, but it will pass. This meal will not make you fat. Tomorrow, you can eat light to offset the meal. You will be fine."

I talk to myself as long as it takes, as many times as it takes, until the urge to purge goes away.

Being honest with your desire to binge, purge, or starve will empower you. Tell a friend, counselor, spouse, family member, or your journal how you feel, but be honest. As the chapter's lead quote says, to tell a lie comes with bigger consequences than facing the truth. It may take practice for you to get in touch with your truth. Maybe you've hidden it from yourself for so long, you no longer know what it is.

Do you allow yourself to eat or do you eat too much?

_____

Why?

_____

_____

_____

What do you feel when you eat, overeat or don't eat?

_____

_____

_____

How do you feel after you eat or binge?

_____

_____

_____

_____

What thoughts go through your head?

_____

_____

_____

_____

Do you play with your food instead of eat?

_____

Why?

_____

_____

_____

_____

Are you afraid to eat?

_____

What do you think would happen if you ate?

_____

_____

_____

What would you tell a friend in your situation?

_____

_____

_____

_____

Do you feel like throwing up after you eat?

_____

What were you feeling before you ate?

_____

_____

_____

_____

Think about your inner self, and what it thinks, feels, and wants.

What are you saying inside?

_____

_____

_____

_____

Can you say those things out loud to yourself?

_____

Is there anything you wish you could say to someone else?

_____

_____

_____

_____

RECOVERY LESSON #14:

Find the humor

> "Humor is mankind's greatest blessing."
> ~*Mark Twain*

My husband gives me gifts of many kinds, but my favorite gift of all is his sense of humor. He shows me how to find the funny in almost any situation and makes me laugh many times a day.

It helps that I *get* his humor. We are more often on the same wavelength than not, and that brings us together. He has suffered much in his life and has learned to use humor to cope. I lost my sense of humor somewhere along the way in my journey, and I forgot how to laugh, and he helped me to remember how. When you are laughing, anger, pain, or resentment takes a pause.

You can't laugh and be angry at the same time. You can stop laughing and be angry. Or sad. Or resentful. However, you cannot experience both emotions simultaneously because genuine laughter happens from an emotion that is opposite of the others.

We live in a broken world, full of harsh realities. Injecting humor will lighten any situation, connect you with others, and make you feel better. Ever laugh at someone because they were laughing, even if you didn't know what made them laugh? Laughter is contagious and releases feel good hormones, making us happier.

Research shows that children laugh up to three hundred times per day. The average grown up? Fourteen times a day. That's a big difference. What if we could up our laugh quota daily, say, by five to ten times more a day?

Get creative. Maybe being around children, or people with a good sense of humor, could get your belly rolling. Perhaps watching something funny or reading silly jokes.

The more you laugh, the more you want to laugh. Why else would we pay to see a stand-up comic or a funny movie? Because we want to laugh.

What would it feel like if you laughed like a five-year-old today? And the next day, and the next? When I managed a sales team, I used humor to help them deal with their stress. I knew it helped me, so I was certain sharing it in the workplace couldn't hurt. To keep morale up, I'd post or email them silly Dad jokes during stressful times. My team members would laugh and thank me. The stupider the jokes, the better they liked them.

There have been times in my life when I couldn't laugh. I was so depressed or distraught that laughter was not possible. After one particular season with no laughter, I realized laughter is a gift. Hard times in life helped me to see the value of laughter and now, whenever I have a chance to laugh, especially at myself, I take full advantage of it. I laugh over the smallest things.

This morning as I was making breakfast, a hair fell onto the plate I was using, and I flung it away. The hair had a dab of butter on it and it clung to the side of the cupboard. A yellow glob of butter with a hair sticking out of it struck me as hilarious, and I had a good chuckle before wiping it up. If there had been a five-year-old in the house, we'd probably still be laughing.

Questions to ask yourself:

Am I laughing every day?

How many times a day do I laugh?

What makes me laugh?

_____

_____

How could I get myself to laugh more?

_____

_____

_____

What would my life like look like if I laughed more?

_____

_____

_____

Explore the possibilities, and then go find something or someone that makes you laugh. Laughter will help you cope with challenging situations and will play a big part in your recovery.

RECOVERY LESSON #15:

Create new rules

)|●|(

> "I had too many rules for myself,
> so I did my best to rewrite them."
> **~Cynthia Star**

Ever dream of rewriting the rules? At school, church, or work? If you were in charge, what rules would you change?

People with eating disorders have a lot of rules. There's a list of do's and don'ts, of cans and can'ts, and of wills and won'ts. Each list grows like a long road that never ends. At least mine did. I still catch myself following self-imposed rules, but I have learned to question my rules, and to rewrite them.

Remember the game you might have played as a child about not stepping on the sidewalk cracks because it would break your mother's back? That's about how silly my rules were. Yet,

I clung to them like lint on a wool sweater- until I challenged their validity.

Just this week, I realized I'd stopped eating bananas because of their sugar and carbohydrate content. They were on my mental list of *can't haves*. I didn't even realize this list still existed. It's a much smaller list than I used to have, so at least that's progress.

How do such lists start? Rules are good, right? They keep us inside the lines of propriety and set a standard of conduct for us. I looked up the definition for "rule" in the Oxford dictionary, which offered:

One of a set of explicit or understood regulations or principles governing conduct within a particular activity or sphere.

I've thought a lot about the lists I've created for myself- where they came from, and why I made them. When I was honest with myself, I figured when and why I made them. Lists gave me a sense of control. False control, but control, none the less.

When I was growing up, I felt like I had no say or control in my chaotic world, so I resorted to making my own rules, ones which I could make myself follow. I unknowingly created rules to feel secure.

Boundaries, like rules, make us feel safe. We know how far we can go when we can see a clear boundary, and they tell us when we have gone too far, like crossing a scrimmage line.

Rules and boundaries are helpful- are necessary- in sports and games, keeping play both fair and fun.

In dysfunctional families, boundaries between people are often gray or non-existent. The more dysfunctional the family, the blurrier the boundaries are between people. It was not until my college years that I got any sense that I didn't have good personal boundaries.

Since I was late applying to college, I was lucky to get a room in a dorm. I was assigned to a corner room with two other roommates. Corner dorm rooms were larger so that they could house three people. Most dorm rooms had space for only two people, and many of my classmates chose their roommates. I gladly took the third bunk in a corner room and wasn't choosy about my roomies.

I was very familiar with the dynamics of three. I was the youngest of three, and had experienced firsthand the dynamics of living in a two against one pattern. With two people, when there are problems, you are more likely to work things out, because it's only you working with one other person. When a third wheel gets added, the propensity for two people to join against one takes hold. That kind of drama played out in my college dorm room. My two roommates joined up against the one of me. There were valid reasons they ganged up on me, and looking back, I don't blame them.

My roommates had lived much different lives than I had. Their parents had coddled them, which became apparent by the many phone calls made, sometimes daily, between them and their parents- not to mention the frequent weekend visits they made back home to their families. They came from mid-dle-class homes, which were complete with a dog, a cat, and 2.1 children. On move-in day, I was alone. I had no family to help me, and I arrived to my room with only the possessions I could carry in the back seat of a car I'd bought myself.

My roommates, however, were both ushered into our room by their parents, siblings, and grandparents, and each brought huge carts stacked with everything anyone could want or need to make a dorm room comfortable. With so much in common, the two of them became fast friends, and I was the odd girl out.

Where I came from, you shared from your abundance, and past friends and I had always lived out of each other's pockets, as we called it, so I assumed my relationships with my dorm mates would be the same way- until one night I awoke to hear the crying of my roommate Ann. She thought I was asleep as she complained over the phone to her mom about me. Want to hear some brutal truth? Overhear a conversation like that.

She sobbed over every detail of my offenses. It's a wonder her mom could stand listening to her wailing. I would have hung up on her quickly into the call. But her behavior was eye opening for me. I must have used her things without asking, like a toaster or a coffee pot, because between sobs that's what I gathered. The one thing I remember that bothered her the most was about her hair brush.

Now, I'm embarrassed to admit that I'd used her brush without asking, but I never thought about the impropriety of that back then. The way she carried on, you would have thought I'd used her underwear or something. Even I know that doing that would have stepped over the line. But I never realized that my simple use of her brush was violating boundaries, and that my lack of personal boundaries was causing her so much grief.

Over the years, I've thought about that conversation and used it as motivation to help me set healthy boundaries. No wonder I created rules of my own. I went from being a person living with few boundaries to a person living by rule lists. The problem is that the rules I set were unrealistic. And the lists I made grew, sometimes daily.

I remember my rule sheet of good and bad foods. On one side of a paper were the good foods I allowed myself to eat, and on the other was a list of foods I couldn't eat. What separated good foods from bad foods were calorie and fat contents. Any anorexic knows the calorie count of every morsel they take in. The list-keeping and calorie counting become an obsession. Like an OCD sufferer, lists get made and re-made until all you do is create lists instead of live life.

The one treat I remember most on my bad list was candy bars. They were forbidden for me to eat. I don't even want a candy bar anymore, so it's no big deal today, but during my eating disorder days, I wanted one candy bar more than anything else. A Butterfinger. Those were my favorite. Before I reached adolescence, I ate a lot of them, but when they made it onto my forbidden list, I never ate another one. And yet, I became obsessed with them. When you deny yourself something, you want it even more. Today, I can eat one of those bite-size candy bars and feel satisfied.

Understanding these behaviors have taken me years to dissect. Working on this book has made me more aware than ever of the unhealthy thought patterns I developed over the years, and has helped me to call many of them into question.

What if I could develop a new set of rules that worked to make me healthy physically and mentally? If I'm so good at making rules, why not make a set that actually works for me? That's the game now. When I discover a self-imposed rule with no validity, like *I can't eat candy bars*, I turn it around to a positive rule.

I did that today with bananas. I love bananas- in cereal, on pancakes, in milkshakes. And I like them at the stage when they just turn yellow, before any brown spots appear. Not too ripe, not too green. When was the last time I ate a banana? Today. When I realized they were on my naughty list.

This is the conversation I had with myself.

"Who says I can't eat bananas?"

"I do."

"Why?"

"Because they are high in sugar and carbohydrates."

"Don't you like bananas?"

"Yes, love them."

"Aren't they good for you?"

"Yes. They contain fiber, potassium, folate, and antioxidants such as vitamin C."

"New rule today, you can eat bananas."

"Who says?"

"Me."

So, I ate banana. I defied myself and my old list and put some banana on top of my pancakes. I did not eat a whole banana, but just part of a banana- eating half of one seemed reasonable for me today. And that is a good start for dispelling such a rule.

If you have created long lists of rules, you can also get rid of those rules- or better yet, you can create new ones like I did with the bananas. If we are so good at creating rules, why not use that power to our advantage?

A first step in this lesson's exercises is to recognize unrealistic rules in your lists. A second step is to challenge those rules, and then replace them with new rules that work to make you healthier. Try it, testing and correcting your list items one rule at a time. Maybe your rules don't apply to food. You can answer the following questions about any rules you have for yourself.

What are some of the rules you've made for yourself?

_____

_____

_____

_____

How long have you had the rule/s?

_____

Do other people follow your rule/s?

_____

Why or why not?

_____

_____

Do you add to your list of rules?

_____

How often do you add more rules?

_____

Is there a rule that you want to get rid of?

_____

Did you make the rule/s you want to get rid of?

_____

If you made the rule/s, why do you think you made that rule?

_____

_____

Could you change the rule?

_____

What would the new rule be?

_____

How did it feel to change a rule?

_____

_____

_____

_____

Is there another rule you would like to change?

_____

How would you change the rule?

_____

What would happen if you got rid of or changed another rule?

_____

_____

_____

_____

The possibilities are endless. The only rule about rules I have now is *have fun ridding yourself of self-imposed rules and changing the rules.* I make it a game, defy myself, and get to eat bananas!

Below are a few "good" rules that I follow. Depending on your circumstances, I suggest you consider adding these to your list of rules.

1. Weigh yourself no more than once a week (less is better). If you are anorexic or obsessed with your weight, this one is important for you to follow.

2. Do not keep foods in the house that might trigger a binge. Know what sets off a binge/purge session and avoid having such things in your cupboards or refrigerator. Ask those around you to keep such fare away from you and not to bring it in your house/space. If you are anorexic, this rule is NOT meant for you. Your new rules must be designed to HELP and encourage you to start eating.

3. It only takes once. Whenever I am tempted to purge (and I still am tempted sometimes), I remind myself that just one slip would put me back into the vicious binge/purge cycle. You may still be trying to break the purging cycle, if so, this one might not be a rule for you, but an encouragement to yourself: *Every day and every meal that I don't purge, is one step closer to being free of my disorder.* If you are an anorexic, it might help to tell yourself something like this: *One more bite or meal than yesterday will help me get better.*

4. Remind yourself daily of how far you have come.

RECOVERY LESSON #16:

Connect with food

> "Our food is one of the most intimate connections we
> make with the earth."
> ~*Gene Bauer*

As a young girl growing up on a farm, I connected with my food daily by feeding and caring for the animals, and collecting their produce (so to speak) when milking a cow, or feeding the chickens and gathering their eggs. Life and death are a natural part of living on a farm, and so is reproduction. Each aspect of life is lived out before your eyes, and you deal with each phase as a natural part of life. Animals breed, give birth, live out their days, and often die in front of you. Living on a farm taught me respect as I connected with the animals in my care.

I also learned to respect my food sources. That may sound weird if you don't know where your food comes from, or how it gets on your table. If you eat meat, eggs, or dairy, it comes from an animal. And that animal sacrifices something for us to partake of a meal, either with its life or its produce (milk, cheese or eggs).

On the farm, I was the keeper of the baby pigs. One of my jobs was to nurse runts (small or weak piglets) back to life. Many runts died in my hands, gasping for breath. An early spring storm might catch us by surprise and if a sow (female pig) gave birth outside instead of in the farrowing barn (a special structure designed to house sows and their babies), it often led to dead or dying piglets. I learned to use warm water in order to revive piglets quickly. There I would be, leaning beside a bathtub of newborn baby pigs, caring for them like they were my own. I loved to watch their cold white skin turn pink and cheery before my eyes. Soon their tails were wiggling, and they were grunting happily.

It didn't take me long to spot the ones past saving, though. I knew the sign of a piglet's impending death and I called it the death gasp. I could tell a pig was done for by the way it gasped for air. No amount of warm water or love would save one that reached this stage. It made me sad to lose even one piglet, but there was no time to spare on them, because the ones that survived needed attention.

I was never particularly fond of pigs once they left my nursery, but I respected them, and the living they provided for us. When the freezer filled up in the fall with fresh pork chops, bacon and ham, I felt grateful to the animal.

A major step in recovery is to reconnect with food at its source. Instead of seeing it as something outside of ourselves, a foreigner to be feared, we can learn to connect, respect and be grateful for it. You may not live on a farm or even be close to one, but there are ways to connect with your food.

Farmers markets have become popular in many areas of the country, allowing consumers to meet growers face-to-face. If you have never been to such a market, why not research your area to see if there is one near you? It might surprise you how much you enjoy the atmosphere, conversation, and down-to-earth feeling that thrives in such places. They often also feature music, artisans of all sorts, and superb food- not fast food, but home-grown, home-cooked, authentic fare. You could attend a farmers market with a few questions ready to ask the merchants so that you might better understand the work it takes for them to grow and produce the offerings they are selling.

Or perhaps there are farms near you that give tours or allow you to take part (even picking your own pumpkin) in the food-to-table process.

Most of the vendors you meet are proud of their products and will gladly answer your questions and elaborate if you ask additional questions. Your goal is to connect with your food, at its source, so you learn to view it in a new way. What are some questions you could ask the grower?

No matter how long I live, the miracle of putting a seed in dirt and watching it produce food or a flower delights me. I can't get over it. To the naked eye, a seed looks lifeless. But when you put it in the soil and add water and sunshine, a miracle happens. Who knew something so beautiful or tasty would appear from this lifeless form?

Have you ever planted anything?

Why not try it?

It doesn't have to be a large undertaking. Set and seed an herb container on your windowsill. Plant one or two potted tomato plants in your yard that you can care for. Set up a small container garden on your patio and raise flowers there that would make you smile. Or simply raise an air plant or a cactus in a pot.

Dirt has magic powers. Not only does it nourish plants, but it can also nourish your soul. Getting your hands dirty does something for us within. It creates a connection between us and the earth that might surprise you. Caring for an animal, a plant, or a flower also gets you outside of yourself and puts your focus elsewhere.

Give yourself permission to fail before you begin. It's ok if the plant or flower dies; you will learn to care for it better the next time. You may also find you have a hidden green thumb talent. For instance, I kill air plants and cactus, but orchids (very challenging) flourish for me. I lost a couple of beautiful orchids before I learned idiosyncrasies about raising them. Had I given up after my early losses, I would not know the pride of watching my orchids bloom year after year. I get excited when the smallest changes occur with each plant.

Watching an orchid grow is like watching a silent movie, and you must watch it carefully to see its story unfolding before you. Months will pass and the smallest growth will occur. A new leaf, root, or the telltale sign of a flower appears with no fanfare. If you are not paying attention, it will catch you by surprise. I have learned through observation to recognize what is happening with my orchids. A leaf turns yellow and dies isn't necessarily bad. Usually, it means the plant has decided it needs the energy to flower or to grow more roots. A nubby green shoot may be a root or a flower. Experience has taught me to know the difference, but it took years of watching these plants for me to discern such things. Now, I know my orchids well, what they need, what they like or dislike, and how to help them thrive.

Having a connection with food, and the earth that it comes from, grounds us in a way that no modern invention or technology can provide. Strong roots are essential for healthy plants- and for healthy people. Digging in the dirt, watching a sprout poke its head out for the first time, and tasting a fresh tomato off the vine may be quintessential to your recovery. It may seem like a silly lesson, but this connection may be just what you need to grow roots of your own that hold you steady through the storms of life.

Our society has recognized how disconnected we are from our food sources, and farmers markets and the farm-to-table (or fork-to-table) movement sprang up quickly in answer to this dilemma. These markets are now popular in many areas throughout the United States. Farm-to-table is a social movement which promotes serving local food at restaurants and school cafeterias, preferably with direct acquisition of food by preparers from the grower. Local farmers, ranchers, wineries, breweries, or fisheries offer their goods in various ways that ensure consumers know the origin of each food. Such channels provide a connection between vendors and the community, and help support small-scale farmers or growers.

Have you ever eaten at a restaurant that serves local fare? This would be another way to connect with your food. The menu typically provides information about the growers' names and the local origins of each meal. The staff should also be knowledgeable about their menu and be able to tell you of the connection between a local source and the food on your plate.

There are also many books on the subject of food connection that might interest you- from memoirs of life on a farm to cookbooks, to stories that focus on how you can eat to flourish. Most of us have become removed from our food sources and how foods get to our table. The goal in this lesson is to connect you to the food you eat in a new way.

Questions to ask yourself:

What is one thing I could do to connect with my food/source?

Are there any farmers markets in my area?

_____

Where are they located?

_____

Could I plan to attend?

_____

Is there someone I could invite to go with me?

_____

What are some questions I might ask the vendors?

_____

_____

_____

_____

What interesting things or people did I see?

_____

_____

_____

Were there things I saw that surprised me?

_____

Would I like to go again?

_____

What did it feel like to talk to the vendors?

_____

_____

_____

Did I learn something new?

_____

_____

_____

Have I ever planted anything?

_____

Why or why not?

_____

_____

_____

What would I like to plant?

_____

_____

_____

How do I start?

_____

_____

_____

_____

What do I need?

_____

_____

_____

_____

Do the plants look different from what I imagined?

_____

What does dirt/soil feel like?

_____

What does it smell like?

_____

Do I like to grow things?

_____

_____

Why or why not?

_____

_____

_____

RECOVERY LESSON #17:

Let food nourish your soul

> "Food for the body is not enough. There must be food
> for the soul."
> ~*Dorothy Day*

Somewhere in my life, I stopped allowing food to nourish me. It became an enemy. What I needed to do was to make it my friend again. But had I spent so many years fighting with it. How was that possible?

Remember, in the first part of my book, I told the story of Welch's grape juice and the memory it invokes for me? It's a wonderful memory that connects me to my dad when I felt loved. Just the scent or sight of Welch's grape juice transports me back in time and reminds me of how food once nourished my soul. As part of my recovery, I use positive memories from my childhood to heal my relationship with food.

Example: One such childhood memory I have is of Quaker instant oatmeal. Then, a box contained eight packets of yummy goodness, and the maple brown sugar kind was my favorite. You'd just add hot water to the packet contents in a bowl and stir. Instant oatmeal was simple enough for us kids to fix on our own, and growing up, my brothers and I enjoyed this treat before heading out to play in the snow or to warm up when we returned half-frozen. It felt like a warm hug on a wintry day.

Recently, a whiff of the maple flavoring reminded me of how much I had loved that treat, so I used my recollection as a way to create a good feeling towards this food as an adult. But I also learned the dry packets I loved as a kid contain much sugar, which could trigger my addiction to sweets. Did you know there have been studies done that show sugar can be more addictive than cocaine? Nobody had to tell me that. I discovered it while standing at the counter as a teenager, making chocolate chip cookies. Studies conducted on rats have revealed that, given the choice, they prefer consuming sugar-sweetened water over cocaine. Below is a quote from that study which is posted online if you care to read the entire article.

"Intense Sweetness Surpasses Cocaine Reward"

By: Magalie Lenoir, Fuschia Serre, Lauriane Cantin, and Serge H AhmedBernhard Baune, Academic Editor

Published on The National Library of Medicine website at www.ncbi.nlm.nih.gov

"We speculate that the addictive potential of intense sweetness results from an inborn hypersensitivity to sweet tastants. In most mammals, including rats and humans, sweet receptors evolved in ancestral environments poor in sugars and are thus not adapted to high concentrations of sweet tastants. The supranormal stimulation of these receptors by sugar-rich diets, such as those now widely available in modern societies, would generate a supranormal reward signal in the brain, with the potential to override self-control mechanisms and thus to lead to addiction."

~ Published online 2007 Aug 1

No wonder young me couldn't stop eating the cookie dough! The reward my brain received from sugar got me addicted, and kept me addicted. If you have a "sweet tooth", or an addiction to sugary foods like I did, your struggle is not just about managing your eating disorder, but also a much stronger addiction cycle. It turns out, our brains are wired to love the sweet stuff, so our fight to resist its pull is real.

The only way I keep that pleasure powder from triggering a binge is to avoid sugar. I once spent three months (ninety days) without sugar to break its hold on me. I had no fruit, no alcohol, and no sugar of any kind. Now, when I eat sweets, it takes very little to satisfy me. One piece of high-quality dark chocolate is enough to satisfy my sweets craving. Intense sweets that once tasted delightful now taste sickening to me. My sweet tooth can creep up on me if I indulge it a little over time. A sweet bite here and taste there leave me wanting more, so I guard myself carefully.

You may not need such drastic measures to overcome an addiction to sweets, but being aware of the power it can hold over you is a big step in recovery. Usually, the more sweets you eat, the more you want.

My challenge became how to create a nutritious, low-sugar version of my beloved childhood treat, instant oatmeal, which fed my body and soul. I used organic oats, real maple flavoring, raw pecans, and a touch of maple syrup, and with a little milk and my favorite spoon, my recipe transported me back in time. I became the happy little girl I used to be, enjoying a bowl of oatmeal, and I savored every bite, which created a positive association for me with this food. I also told myself, "I deserve to eat food that tastes good and fuels my body. "

The reason I go back to my childhood to conjure up positive memories of food is for two reasons.

Number one, young children do what comes naturally. They eat when they're hungry and they stop when they're full, and then they go off to play with no second thoughts. They go through picky stages, ravenous stages, or hunger strikes (when they are sick). I needed to get back in touch with my intrinsic rhythm for eating, and childhood memories reminded me of what that felt like, when food for me wasn't an addiction or a crutch.

That is the state of being I reach for now each day- to be in tune with my body, listening to it as I did when I was a child. Being able to do this takes practice, focus, and determination.

I often ask myself before I eat, "Am I really hungry or am I trying to feed an unmet need?"

If I'm genuinely hungry, I eat. If not, I try to find the unmet need. You will know you are trying to feed an unmet need when you binge or overeat regularly. Everyone overeats occasionally. We live in a land of abundance, so for most of us, it's easy to do. But overeating to fill an emptiness differs from stuffing yourself in an occasional overindulgence. You can never eat enough to fill an emotional emptiness, because food isn't what you need- it's what you are using to fill an emptiness inside. You can never eat enough food to feel emotionally full.

When I was bingeing, I felt disconnected from my body, and I mindlessly shoved food into my mouth, unaware of what I was feeling physically or emotionally. My eating was an escape from reality. And that is how it became an addiction.

Sometimes I don't eat for part of a day until I feel super hungry, just to remind myself what hunger feels like. Food tastes much better when you are genuinely hungry, but I am also careful not to let myself get so hungry that I scarf everything in sight, or eat too fast. Other times, I wake up famished and eat shortly after I arise. When you are in tune with your body and emotionally full, you will know when to eat and when to stop. With practice, you can learn to be in tune with your body's signals.

The second reason I use childhood memories is to bring up a feeling of being nurtured, which also helps me to develop a positive association with food. Did you notice I used a favorite spoon to eat my oatmeal?

Why would that be important?

Do you have a favorite cup? Most people do, because a favorite cup makes things taste better. It feels good in your hands, or maybe you love the color or shape of its handle. It's easy to hold, is the size you prefer, and makes you feel good about drinking coffee, tea, or any beverage.

Did you have a favorite spoon, plate, or cup as a child? I can't recall one specific cutlery piece or saucer, but I remember how it felt to be nurtured, and it was also through foods I was given. My mother was a nurturer, so it's easy for me to remember times I felt that way- like when she made me eggs Benedict on toast after a lengthy illness, and it was the only meal I'd eat for days. I also remember how much I loved chicken pot pies, served hot in a metal tin at my favorite babysitter's house. I still love chicken pot pie, and I recently treated myself to that feel-good meal. It tasted as good as I remembered and left me feeling warm and cozy.

I have a favorite spoon that makes me feel that way. It's a hand-crafted wooden spoon that is gently curved and fits my hand perfectly. It was a gift from my son-in-law, and when I eat with it, I feel loved and nurtured. I moved recently and forgot about it for a time, but upon discovering my lost treasure, I returned it to its place of honor on my counter and resumed using it daily.

If you are bingeing, purging, or overeating, your lesson in this chapter is to find the unmet need or unfaced feelings that you are trying to feed (or escape from) through eating, which may take some time. Keeping a journal will help you recognize patterns, triggers, and unfaced feelings. Instead of beating yourself up verbally, be gentle with yourself and acknowledge you are a work in progress. You goal is not to win or lose, but to uncover the layers of emotional issues so that you can deal with them.

If you are an anorexic, struggling to eat, have a list of forbidden foods, or feel anxious when you eat, this lesson is to help you get past your fear and gain a positive connection with food.

Here are some questions to ask:

Do you remember a time when food nourished your soul?

_____

_____

_____

What did that feel like?

_____

_____

_____

What dish/es transport you back to that time?

_____

Do I allow food to nourish my soul?

_____

Why or why not?

_____

_____

_____

What would it look like to let food nourish my soul?

_____

_____

_____

Do you have a favorite item (dish/spoon/cup) that might connect you to a happy time?

_____

Would it feel good to use that favorite item?

_____

Are there meals/food that I could create (or recreate) that would feel nourishing to my body and soul?

_____

_____

_____

Is that meal/food going to trigger my sugar addiction (if you have one)?

_____

If so, how could I create a version that would be satisfying for me without triggering my addiction?

_____

_____

If I made that meal/food, will I allow myself to enjoy it?

_____

Do I feel like I deserve to be nourished?

_____

Why or why not?

_____

_____

_____

Do you remember when you didn't binge, purge or starve yourself?

_____

What did that feel like?

_____

_____

Are you eating to fill an unmet emotional need?

What unmet need/s are you trying to fill?

RECOVERY LESSON #18:

Dine well

> "One cannot think well, love well, sleep well, if one
> has not dined well."
> ~ *Virginia Woolf*

What does it mean to dine well? Only you can answer that question for yourself, but I will share what it means to me, and how this lesson has been instrumental in my recovery. For me, dining well means to eat the best foods possible in a manner that is pleasing to my senses.

I like to cook and use organic, free range, and antibiotic free foods when possible. Throughout the years, I've gathered healthy recipes for a variety of dishes- gourmet recipes for main dishes, soups, salads, and dressings, replacing sugar-ladened desserts with nutritious alternatives, because when I dine, I want the most nutritious and delicious meals possible. When food feeds your body and soul, it becomes an experience, not just a meal. And that is the goal of this lesson.

After a satisfying meal, you feel satiated. This differs from bingeing. When I binged, I would stand at the kitchen counter, stuffing my face as fast as I could and disconnect from my feelings. Dining well is being present while you are eating. For me, it includes finding the recipes, shopping for the ingredients, setting an attractive table and sitting down to dine.

I love fresh flowers, so I buy them when I can, or use artificial ones as a centerpiece. Colorful place mats, shiny silverware (or my favorite spoon) and fancy plates set the mood for a satisfying meal. The old saying, "We eat with our eyes," is true, so I try to make my meal visually appealing as well as tasty.

I have been practicing the art of dining well for years, but when I met my husband six years ago, I changed my habits a little at a time until I stopped cooking for myself. He is a picky eater and rarely eats what I fix. It seemed like too much trouble to cook for myself (my belief) so I slid into some bad habits, like eating more processed and frozen foods.

My mistake was changing my behavior to suit him. He never asked me to change what or how I prepared for meals. I did it to myself. What I unknowingly did was alter my relationship with food, and while writing this book, I realized how far I'd gone. I got lazy and stopped creating healthy meals for myself (which is ok to do once in a while, but not regularly).

So, I made myself some new rules:

1) Set an attractive table for every meal with placemats, flowers and cloth napkins.

2). Sit down, square on your chair, when you eat.

3.) Give thanks for your food.

5). Soak in the aroma of your dish.

6.) Pay attention to taste, texture, colors of your food.

4.) Eat slowly, enjoying every bite.

I've returned to cooking several meals a week, digging up my favorite recipes. I invite my husband to partake with me, but I have no expectations that he will accept. If he does, we dine together, but if he declines, that doesn't keep me from enjoying my meal. If I have leftovers that are not eaten within a few days, I freeze the rest for later.

I empowered myself to eat well by adopting new rules.

Here are some questions to ask:

What would it look like for me to dine well?

_____

_____

_____

Could I dine well at every meal?

_____

Think about your favorite restaurant. What do you appreciate about being there?

_____

_____

_____

Could I create an inviting atmosphere for myself?

_____

What would that look like?

_____

_____

_____

What would it look like to create a similar dish from my favorite restaurant?

_____

What are the steps I would take if company was coming for dinner?

_____

_____

_____

Have I ever done those things for myself?

_____

Why or why not?

_____

_____

_____

What would inviting myself to dine look like?

_____

_____

_____

What healthy rules could I establish for eating well?

_____

_____

_____

_____

Here is another idea. You could play a game with yourself while learning what it means to dine well. Take something simple and turn it into the extraordinary.

Example: I've started turning the ordinary into the extraordinary, like my coffee. I use the best tasting (sugar-free) coffee creamer I can get, and I add vanilla extract, cinnamon, and nutmeg on top to turn my plain cup of Joe into a special treat I enjoy every day. Because I'm worth it. It is fun coming up with creative ways to turn the mundane in life into the sublime.

The more you enjoy your food and drink, the more satisfying it becomes. You can add texture, color, spice or flavor to an ordinary meal (or a cup of coffee) to turn it into a tasty delight. You can set a fabulous table, use fine china, or just use a favorite spoon or dish. The goal in this lesson is to encourage you to dine well and feed your soul.

Think about turning something as simple as a cup of tea or coffee into an experience for your soul.

What ordinary experience could I turn into the extraordinary?

_____

How does the ordinary taste?

_____

How does it taste after I add an extraordinary flare?

_____

Did I enjoy the extraordinary more than the ordinary?

_____

What would it be like if I dined well at every meal?

_____

_____

_____

RECOVERY LESSON #19:

Celebrate everything

> "When we fail to acknowledge and celebrate small victories, we get discouraged and the flame inside us starts to dwindle."
> *~Unknown*

How do you overcome an eating disorder? One bite at a time. Whether you overeat, undereat, binge, purge or starve, the only way to recover is one bite at a time.

I picture myself climbing a ladder. Some days I step up the ladder, some days I step back down. If I keep taking steps up, even if I go down a few, eventually, I will get to the top. How long that takes does not matter to me, only that I keep reaching for the top. As long as I'm on the ladder, I'm making progress. Even if I don't move at all.

Fear of failure. That's what drove me into my eating disorder. It's also what kept me there. The smallest failure became self-defeating. Win or lose, that's all I knew. If I binged or purged, I was a failure and the self-hatred took over, keeping me in a vicious cycle.

One step down the ladder and would I beat myself up. Would I beat up a friend for taking a step back on their ladder? Heck no, I'd encourage them to keep going. I'd praise them for every small step up they took.

A wise old man once told me, "Celebrate everything!" He'd lived long enough to know life goes fast and you never know when it might end, so celebrate while you can.

Examples: Fresh flowers on the table make me happy, so I often buy them for myself. The smallest victory is cause for a fresh bouquet. If I had the space in our house, I would treat myself to a new plant regularly because I love them, and marvel at all the different species. I also reward myself by allowing myself extra time for a creative outlet.

Think of ways you can celebrate even the smallest victory.

Grab a cup of your favorite coffee, get silly stickers to place on your journal, or a new pen that you'd love to write with. It doesn't have to be extravagant, as long as you take time to celebrate your accomplishments, and simply life around you.

I have a friend I particularly enjoy being with. We keep a list of things to celebrate, no matter how small they might be. She is my outdoorsy friend and enjoys hiking, snowshoeing or walking along the river. After an adventure, we dine together, rarely at the same place twice, sharing a meal and a toast to cheer our achievements. Her company makes me happy and I feel content long after one of our friendship dates.

If you want to heal your relationship with food, learn to celebrate every step forward and treat every step back graciously, like you would with a friend. Food did not become your enemy overnight, and it will not become your friend in one day. It will be a process that takes as long as it takes.

Questions to ask:

Do I celebrate my successes?

_____

Why/Why not?

_____

_____

_____

Do I think it's ok to celebrate accomplishments?

_____

How could I celebrate more?

_____

Do I celebrate others' accomplishments?

_____

How does that make me feel?

_____

_____

_____

Do I believe I'm worthy of celebrating?

_____

Why or why not?

_____

_____

_____

_____

What would it look like if I celebrated every small step I took forward?

_____

_____

_____

What is one success (no matter how small) that I could celebrate today?

_____

How did it feel to celebrate?

_____

_____

_____

Could I do that again?

_____

Here are some ideas for celebrating:

Give yourself a gold star or a fun sticker.

Let someone give you a gold star or fun sticker.

Clap your hands.

Smile at yourself in the mirror.

Tell someone about your success and let them clap for you.

Throw confetti.

Blow a paper horn.

Draw a smiley face.

Toast yourself.

Tell yourself how well you did.

Let someone else tell you how well you did.

Ask someone to tell you how well you did.

Throw your arms up over your head.

Dance around.

Skip.

Jump up and down.

Give a thumbs up.

Make or buy a party hat and wear it.

Wear a tiara.

Make a banner.

Sing a song.

Play a musical instrument

Write/draw something celebratory on a chalkboard.

Why not set a creative date with yourself? One day a week, allot time for an adventure. Visit a museum, an art gallery, a local shop or lie beneath the clouds on a spring day. Buy a coloring book, a sketch pad or gather rocks. Dust off your imagination and get inspired. You decide what might spur your creativity. Look around for inspiration and ask the child inside, what would delight them?

RECOVERY LESSON #20:

Surround yourself
with healthy people

> "The people you surround yourself with influence your behaviors, so choose friends who have healthy habits."
> ~*Dan Buettner*

The tricky part about an eating disorder is, unlike other addictions, you can't just stop eating. You must continue to navigate food for the rest of your life. If you want to have a healthy relationship with food, surround yourself with people that have good eating habits. They will show you what it looks like to be friends with food.

Think of groups you know, and the people that each attracts. Someone that wants to learn a skill they don't have seeks out those who can teach them that skill. Positive or negative habits rub off on us, so choosing to spend time with people that are positive role models is imperative for your recovery.

A group of anorexics housed together will soon become better anorexics. The same would go for a house of bulimics, or bingers. Do not underestimate the competitive nature of an eating disorder, especially in an anorexic. Anorexics will often garner tips from one another and then use them to outdo each other.

That's not to say you can't have a friend or family member around that has unhealthy eating habits, but spending too much time with that kind of person will affect you, either positively or negatively. If I wanted to learn to invest, paint, write a book, or skateboard, I would seek or hire those that could teach me. And when I learned everything that I could garner from them, I'd find someone else who could teach me more. Who you hang with matters.

If your family or friends don't have healthy eating habits, find people that do and eat with them. They will teach you what a healthy relationship with food looks like.

Example: Life growing up on a farm was hectic. There was so much to do! My mom was busy outside most of the time. She was an excellent cook, but rarely had time to teach me, so I spent a good deal of time teaching myself how to cook. I developed poor eating habits, like standing at the counter bingeing on cookie dough. One night, I visited a friend's house for dinner and the stark contrast between my house and hers left a lasting impression in my memory.

When we arrived after school, her mom greeted us at the door, offered us snacks on a tray, and informed us we could relax after doing our homework. Later, she called us into the kitchen to help with dinner preparation. My job was to peel the carrots. I'd never peeled carrots before and I was confused. We just washed the carrots before eating them at my house. I was too embarrassed to ask what was expected, so I took the initiative and peeled the carrots vigorously. By the time I got done, there was not much left but twigs. I proudly handed her the plate of peeled carrots. It's funny looking back, but at the time I didn't know any different. My friend's mom was very gracious. She smiled and thanked me for a job well done. The whole family gathered around the dinner table, held hands as we said grace, and politely handed the food around family style. This was a normal day at their house, not a holiday or special occasion.

That one afternoon revealed a new world to me- that there was a family dynamic that differed from my own, and it was an example of a healthy one for me. Imagine if I ate at that house day after day, how my relationship with food would have developed differently.

Spending time with others that have healthy habits, not just related to food, will rub off on you, so choose wisely your company. If you don't know what healthy habits look like, ask your counselor, therapist, or study other cultures that treat food with respect and gratitude. The healthier you become, the healthier you will want to get, and the easier it will be to recognize healthy habits in others.

Questions to ask yourself:

What does it look like when people have a healthy relationship with food?

_____

_____

_____

Do the people I spend the most time with have a healthy relationship with food?

_____

Do I know anyone that I could eat with that could teach me how to have a healthy relationship with food?

_____

Are there any of my friends that don't have a healthy relationship with food?

_____

How much time do I spend with those friends?

_____

Is the time I spend with others teaching me good or bad habits?

_____

What would it look like to spend time with someone who has healthy eating habits?

_____

_____

_____

RECOVERY LESSON #21:

Practice gratitude

> "Gratitude is the ability to experience life as a gift. It liberates us from the prison of self-preoccupation."
> *~John Ortberg*

You are probably thinking, what does gratitude have to do with overcoming an eating disorder? It is no mistake that I saved this lesson for last. **This one lesson, if learned well, will change your life for the better.**

The practice of gratitude puts our focus on what we have, instead of what we don't have. It gets us outside of ourselves, our problems, and away from self-pity. It releases a positive energy, and the more you practice gratitude, the more grateful you become.

I have learned to find something to be grateful for in almost every situation. And I call it my "attitude of gratitude."

Example: Parking is a problem in my city of Albuquerque. Almost everywhere I go, it's hard to find a parking spot. My "attitude of gratitude" started one day when I not only found an open spot near my destination, but it was located under a tree. Summer lasts a long time in New Mexico, so competition is high for shaded parking areas. I was so excited to find that primo spot, I gave thanks and did a little happy dance. The next time I went out, I found a parking spot right up near the establishment. I repeated my gratitude practice as I went inside.

Now, I almost always find a good parking spot, even in crowded situations. I confidently search the lot, sending out good vibes, and an open spot usually appears. It's not magic or an act of God, but energetically, the positive vibes I put out there seem to return. All I know is, the more grateful I am, the better things I receive.

It takes the same energy to grumble and complain as it does to be grateful. But the results of gratitude have far superior results. There is always something to be grateful for. It might take a while to see it, but the good in any situation is there if you look hard enough. Your attitude will shift positively, one grateful moment at a time, until gratitude will become your norm.

My friend has a saying that I live by.

"What you focus on expands."

Years ago, I had my first and only traffic accident. Another driver rear-ended me and I suffered severe whiplash. Since then, I've been to a chiropractor, a pain specialist, and received dry needling and physical therapy, but the pain persists on my left side. I still experience muscle spasms, headaches, and it affects my life daily. Because of my pain and suffering, I received a small settlement from the other driver's insurance. After I paid my medical bills, there wasn't much left of the settlement, but I used that money to put a small down payment on a house. The timing was perfect because interest rates and house prices were low at that moment. That house has almost doubled in value in only 6 years, and it has provided me with a happy home and will allow me to retire earlier than I planned.

Every time I'm tempted to complain about my neck pain, I think about how blessed I am to have my house and I give thanks. It would never have been possible for me to buy a house without the accident.

When you focus on the good, the good gets better. If you focus on the bad, it gets worse.

We have a choice many times a day where we put our focus. Where will you put your focus today?

Can you find the good (no matter how small) in a recent unpleasant situation?

Write down five things you are grateful for.

_____ _____

_____

_____

_____

_____

Keep the list and see if you can expand it to ten or even twenty things.

Use your list to feel grateful for one thing every day.

What would it look like to start your own Attitude of Gratitude practice?

_____

_____

_____

Gratitude, in my experience, is the secret to finding happiness. Grateful people find happiness because they focus on the good, and the good expands. Like the Grinch, many peoples' hearts are two sizes too small until they learn that happiness comes from being grateful. Your heart will grow when you practice gratitude. The happier you are, the less power your eating disorder will have over you, until one day, you overcome what you thought was impossible.

Conclusion

When food has control over us, we have no control over food. Our eating disorders give us a false sense of control, but in reality, we have no control until we make a shift to a healthy relationship with food, and ultimately, with ourselves, which usually leads into better relationships with those around us. Good relationships take time to foster, so be patient.

You may not be ready to give up your eating disorder. It is time to be honest with yourself.

Ask yourself:

Am I ready to give up my eating disorder?

_____

Why or why not?

_____

_____

_____

What would make me ready?

_____

_____

_____

Only you can decide when you are ready to complete any or all of the lessons in this book. Recovery starts by asking yourself these questions, though.

If you use your eating disorder as a crutch, an escape, a cry for attention, or a cry for love, it may take more time than you expected to find healing. Explore the hard questions in these chapters a little at a time. When you are ready, you will know it is time to forge ahead.

After all these years, I still re-align my relationship with food when it's necessary. So don't be surprised if you find yourself needing a realignment from time to time.

A big force that drives an eating disorder is the pursuit of per-fection. Ask yourself if you are striving for perfection. What if you gave yourself permission to get C's in life, instead of demanding A's of yourself?

What would that look like?

_____

_____

_____

I am much happier getting a C in life, with an A here or there. I hope you someday you will allow yourself the same.

Be kind to yourself as you go through these lessons. There is some hard work involved. You can be happy and healthy, free of your eating disorder. You just need to believe it as I believe it for you.

There is a woman I see often as I'm driving on a particular street. She speed-walks in all kinds of weather, all times of the day. I'm certain she is anorexic. I recognize the gaunt face, the protruding bones, the drive to exercise, even in inclement weather. My heart hurts for her, and I send her love while I pass her by. My heart hurts for you as well, suffering friend, and I wish you love, healing, and happiness. As long as you draw breath, there is hope for you. In every day, at every meal, every bite can be a new beginning for you if you let it.

What does your life look like without an eating disorder?

_____

_____

_____

_____

_____

Imagine the possibilities and write them down. Every success starts in the mind.

What you think about comes about.

Does it seem impossible to be free of your eating disorder? I believed that too. Now I know it is possible, as I am proof of it.

If I did it, so can you.

I believe you will be free. Keep taking that next step until someday you find yourself at the top of the ladder.

Here is a poem I want to share with you about loving yourself. My hope for you is that you will learn to love the skin you're in.

Love the skin you're in

I want the world to know, it's not about what shows

What means the most lies within,

beneath the layers of your skin.

Red, yellow, black or white,

it fits just right, not too tight

It's uniquely you.

Big or small, fat or thin

It's the skin you was born in

No one gets to choose.

It just ain't fair,

I look like this; I want to look like that.

Who says it's better over there?

You're fair just as you is.

Big or small, short or tall,

God loves us one and all

Some were blessed with so much less

Some seem to have it all

It doesn't really matter;

You're the best of you.

No matter where you're going,

or where you might have been

It's all you're ever gonna get,

so love the skin you're in.

~Cynthia Star

Would you take the time to leave an honest review on Amazon? Reviews help readers find the right books, so thank you!

End Notes

1). Online article cited in Recovery lesson #17 of this book.

"Intense Sweetness Surpasses Cocaine Reward"

By: Magalie Lenoir, Fuschia Serre, Lauriane Cantin, and Serge H Ahmed

Bernhard Baune, Academic Editor

Published online 2007, Aug. 1

Article can be found at: The National Library of Medicine website

2). Online article cited in Part Two: Recovery lesson in this book.

"The Neurobiology of Noshing: Why is it so easy to overeat calorie-rich tasty foods?"

Kash is a member of the UNC Bowles Center for Alcohol Studies

This research was funded by grants from the National Institute on Alcohol Abuse and Alcoholism (NIAAA), The National Institute of Diabetes and Digestive and Kidney Diseases (NIDDK), the North Carolina Biotech Center, and the Swedish Research Council.

If you care to read the article, it can be found at: the UNC Health and UNC School of Medicine website

Published online 2019, April 24

About the Author

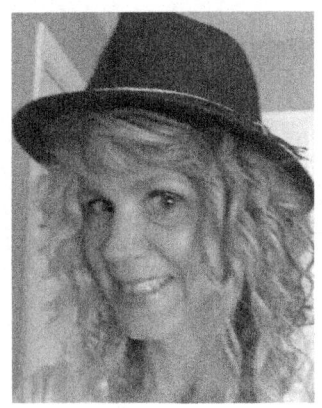

When I was growing up, I read every dog or horse book that I could get my hands on. I loved reading so much that I dreamed of being an author and wrote my first book at age ten. I was lucky enough to grow up on a farm in rural Nebraska, and then spent thirty years in wonderful Wyoming before moving to the Southwest. I now live in Albuquerque, hiking the foothills often while I dream up my next story.

You can check out all my books at www.CynthiaStarBooks.com (know anyone who likes dragons?)

If this book helped you, I'd love to hear about it. Email me at: CynaStar019@gmail.com.

Happiness is always on the other side of fear.

~Margie Johnson